Cognitive Behavior Therapy for Binge Eating Disorder

Riccardo Dalle Grave
Massimiliano Sartirana • Simona Calugi

Cognitive Behavior Therapy for Binge Eating Disorder

Springer

Riccardo Dalle Grave
Department of Eating and Weight Disorders
Villa Garda Hospital
Verona, Italy

Massimiliano Sartirana
Associazione Disturbi Alimentari (ADA)
Verona, Italy

Simona Calugi
Department of Eating and Weight Disorders
Villa Garda Hospital
Garda, Verona, Italy

ISBN 978-3-031-71455-9 ISBN 978-3-031-71456-6 (eBook)
https://doi.org/10.1007/978-3-031-71456-6

This Springer imprint is published by the registered company Springer Nature Switzerland AG
The registered company address is: Gewerbestrasse 11, 6330 Cham, Switzerland

Preface

"Binge eating" is a term first coined by the American physician Albert Stunkard in 1959 to describe the behaviour of a subgroup of patients with obesity[1] who experienced recurrent episodes of excessive and uncontrolled eating. However, it was not until the late 1980s that binge-eating disorder (BED) was recognized as a distinct clinical entity, when some studies on bulimia nervosa discovered a large subgroup of individuals in the population who did not use compensatory behaviours after binge-eating episodes. During the same period, it was observed that about a quarter of individuals seeking treatment for obesity reported recurrent binge-eating episodes but did not suffer from bulimia nervosa.

In 1994, the American Psychiatric Association (APA) included BED as an example of an eating disorder not otherwise specified and provided a list of diagnostic criteria for further study in Appendix B of their fourth Diagnostic and Statistical Manual of Mental Disorders (DSM-IV). Subsequent research confirmed that BED indeed has clinical features that set it apart from bulimia nervosa and obesity, supporting the validity and clinical utility of its diagnosis. These findings resulted in the inclusion of BED as a distinct diagnostic category in the 2013 DSM-5.

Although BED can be seen in individuals within the normal body mass index (BMI, measured in kg/m^2) range, it is more common in those with obesity. Among people seeking treatment for obesity, about 9% meet the DSM diagnostic criteria for BED. However, about 30% of the same population report the presence of

[1] The term "obesity" is used, as defined by the World Health Organization (WHO), when a person has a BMI $\geq$ 30 According to WHO categories for adults over 20 years old, BMI < 18.5 denotes underweight; BMI 18.5–24.9 normal weight; BMI $\geq$ 25 overweight (pre-obesity); and BMI $\geq$ 30 obesity. Some eating disorder organizations have suggested that the terms overweight and obesity be discarded in favour of other, less stigmatizing, more neutral and inclusive terms such as "higher weight individual" or "person with a larger body" without a BMI cutoff. However, as the National Institutes of Health (NIH) style guide has recommended, these terms should be used when writing outside a scientific, clinical, or public health context (or a press release reporting on a clinical study). In a scientific context, "higher body weight" or similar general terms should not be used as synonyms for overweight and obesity. The guide also recommends using "person with obesity", "person affected by obesity", or "person who has obesity" instead of "obese person" or "they are obese". Following the NIH recommendations, we have used the terms "higher weight", "larger body", and "weight" only in the clinical transcripts, while the terms "obesity", "overweight", and "person with obesity" are used in the rest of this book.

binge-eating episodes. Furthermore, BED has been found in about 50% of bariatric surgery candidates with a BMI $\geq$ 50.0.

Over the last 15 years, more than 2,500 articles on BED have been published in international scientific journals, providing us with in-depth information on its main clinical characteristics. The studies conducted to date have also highlighted two problems that complicate treatment. The first of these is that binge eating is maintained by several mechanisms that are heterogeneous and vary from individual to individual, and the second is that available psychological treatments have a limited effect in patients with obesity and BED.

With this in mind, we have devised a specific form of cognitive behaviour therapy (CBT) to help patients with BED interrupt their binge-eating episodes, and, if indicated, achieve healthy weight loss. The aim of this treatment is for such patients to address and overcome the main mechanisms underlying their disorder in a personalized and flexible way. To this end, the treatment incorporates strategies and procedures from two evidence-based psychological interventions: (i) the enhanced version of CBT for eating disorders (also known as CBT-E) and (ii) personalized CBT for obesity (also known as CBT-OB). CBT is the only psychological treatment recommended for eating disorders by the National Institute for Health and Care Excellence (NICE) guidelines for all diagnostic categories of adults and adolescents with eating disorders. It has been particularly effective in reducing binge-eating episodes. Personalized CBT-OB has been demonstrated to help patients with clinical obesity (i.e., when an individual's physical health and or psychosocial functioning is significantly impaired due to obesity) to achieve healthy weight loss in randomized controlled trials and real-world clinical setting studies.

CBT for BED adopts the key principles of CBT-E and personalized CBT-OB, including the collaborative style of therapy, the general structure of the sessions, strategies for encouraging the patient's active participation in the treatment, and an individualized and flexible approach in its content and duration. However, the treatment also includes specific strategies to address the distinctive overeating and dysregulated eating between binge-eating episodes, low activity levels, internalized weight stigma, unrealistic weight goals, and overvaluation of shape and weight that often afflict people with BED associated with clinical obesity.

The treatment is well-suited for both males and females, and patients do not require specific cognitive skills to benefit. It has been designed primarily for individual administration in an outpatient setting for patients at least 16 years of age.

In selected patients with clinical obesity, CBT for BED can also be effectively combined with modern incretin-based weight-loss drugs. These medications have shown remarkable efficacy in promoting weight loss and maintenance. They also play a significant role in preventing type 2 diabetes, reducing cardiovascular disease (CVD) risk factors, and addressing the major complications of clinical obesity. Additionally, they contribute to improving the quality of life and overall well-being of individuals with clinical obesity.

This book is written in the form of a manual for clinicians and is divided into two parts. Part One describes the most up-to-date scientific knowledge on BED and the cognitive-behaviour theory of BED. It then gives an overview of the treatment and how to implement it effectively. Part Two describes the core protocol of CBT for BED. To assist practitioners, the treatment is detailed from the first to the last session, with clinical transcripts and vignettes included to illustrate highlights and strategies for tailoring the intervention to individual patient needs.

This book is recommended for all clinicians who treat people with BED with or without clinical obesity (e.g., psychiatrists, internists, endocrinologists, psychologists, dietitians, nutritionists, nurses, educators, and physical therapists). It is also useful for clinicians (e.g., gynaecologists, endocrinologists, gastroenterologists, haematologists, allergists, psychiatrists, psychotherapists, and psychologists) who, although not working in specialized eating disorder and obesity clinics, are involved in managing the medical and psychiatric comorbidities of BED.

Before we proceed further, we would like to take this opportunity to thank Zafra Cooper for her pioneering work in emphasizing the importance of cognitive processes in maintaining binge-eating episodes and obesity and integrating CBT-E for eating disorders with CBT for obesity. A heartfelt thank you also goes to all our colleagues for their valuable advice that helped improve the treatment. Finally, our special thanks go to the patients we have treated, who have provided fundamental suggestions for perfecting the treatment presented in this book.

Garda, Italy — Riccardo Dalle Grave
Verona, Italy — Massimiliano Sartirana
Garda, Italy — Simona Calugi

Contents

Abbreviations

ACE	Angiotensin-converting enzyme
ADHD	Attention deficit hyperactivity disorder
ARBs	Angiotensin receptor blockers
BED	Binge-eating disorder
BMI	Body mass index
BWLT	Behavioural weight-loss therapy
CBT	Cognitive behaviour therapy
CBT-E	Enhanced cognitive behaviour therapy
CBTgsh	Cognitive behaviour therapy-based self-help
CBT-OB	Cognitive behaviour therapy for obesity
CVD	Cardiovascular disease
DBT	Dialectical behaviour therapy
DPP-4	Dipeptidyl peptidase 4
DSM-5	Diagnostic and Statistical Manual of Mental Disorders
EDEQ	Eating Disorder Examination Questionnaire
EPCL-BED	Eating problem checklist for binge-eating disorder
FDA	Food and Drug Administration
GERD	Gastroesophageal reflux disease
GFR	Glomerular filtration rate
GIP	Glucose-dependent insulinotropic polypeptide
GLP-1	Glucagon-like peptide-1
GLP-1ARs	Glucagon-like peptide-1 receptor agonists
HRQoL	Health-related quality of life
ICD-11	International Classification of Diseases, 11th Revision
IPT	Interpersonal psychotherapy
IUD	Intrauterine device
IWS	Internalized weight stigma
LDX	Lisdexamfetamine
MAFLD	Metabolic dysfunction-associated fatty liver disease
MAOIs	Monoamine oxidase inhibitors
MASH	Metabolic dysfunction-associated steatohepatitis
NICE	National Institute for Health and Care Excellence
NSAIDs	Nonsteroidal anti-inflammatory drugs
NWCR	National Weight Control Registry

OEDs	Other eating disorders
PCOS	Polycystic ovary syndrome
SGLT2	Sodium-glucose transport protein 2
SSRI	Selective serotonin reuptake inhibitor
TCAs	Tricyclic antidepressants
WH	Waist:hip
WHO	World Health Organization

Part I

Introduction & Overview

Binge-Eating Disorder: General Information

1

Abstract

Binge-eating disorder (BED) is characterized by recurrent binge-eating episodes not followed by the regular use of compensatory behaviours. For a diagnosis of BED, these episodes are to occur at least once a week over 3 months and be accompanied by significant distress. Recent data on BED indicates a lifetime prevalence of 0.42% in men and 1.25% in women, 0.85% overall. While it does occur in normal-weight individuals, BED is more prevalent in those with higher weight. It frequently coexists with various psychological problems (e.g., overvaluation of shape and weight in about 50% of cases), mental disorders (e.g., depression, anxiety, substance use, and impulse control issues), and general medical conditions (e.g., cardiometabolic diseases). Psychological treatments, such as cognitive behaviour therapy (CBT), can induce remission in approximately 50–55% of patients with BED. Nonetheless, their impact on weight loss is limited, especially in cases in which BED is associated with clinical obesity. Pharmacological interventions for anxiety and depression have some efficacy in reducing BED symptoms. However, while certain drugs demonstrate promise, they often have significant side effects. Recognizing the need for a treatment to address both binge-eating episodes and the related psychopathology, while also achieving clinically significant weight loss when indicated, a novel approach named "CBT for BED" has been developed. CBT for BED integrates strategies and procedures from enhanced CBT for eating disorders and personalized CBT for obesity.

1.1 Key Features

The main characteristic of binge-eating disorder (BED) is recurrent binge-eating episodes. An episode of binge eating is characterized by both of the following [1]:

R. Dalle Grave et al., *Cognitive Behavior Therapy for Binge Eating Disorder*,
https://doi.org/10.1007/978-3-031-71456-6_1

1. Eating, over a discrete period of time (e.g., within any 2-hour period), an amount of food that is definitely larger than most people would eat in a similar period of time under similar circumstances
2. The sense of lack of control over eating during the episode (e.g., a feeling that one cannot stop eating or control what or how much one is eating)

The weakening of control may not be absolute. For example, an individual may continue eating while the telephone rings, but interrupt it if a family member enters the room. In some cases, there is not an acute sensation of loss of control, but rather a general dysregulated and uncontrolled way of eating [2]. Some individuals completely abandon the attempt to control eating, and therefore do not feel a loss of control of eating. In contrast, other individuals schedule binge-eating episodes. In the latter two cases, the episodes are considered binges if the individual feels unable to do without them.

In BED, eating a large amount of food is associated with loss of control. Such binge-eating episodes are referred to as objective, to distinguish them from subjective binging, in which feeling a loss of control is not actually associated with eating a large amount of food. If loss of control is not present, the terms objective or subjective overeating are used to describe the episode, depending on the amount of food consumed, i.e., large or not, respectively [3]. The different patterns of actual vs. perceived overeating are not mutually exclusive, and people with BED often report both objective and subjective binge-eating episodes that occur in the context of dysregulated and excessive eating.

According to the DSM-5, a diagnosis of BED requires the presence of at least one objective binge-eating episode per week for 3 months associated with marked distress, and at least three of the following features [1]:

- Eating much more rapidly than normal
- Eating until feeling uncomfortably full
- Eating large amounts of food when not feeling physically hungry
- Eating alone because of being embarrassed by how much one is eating
- Feeling disgusted with oneself, depressed, or very guilty after overeating

In addition, the binge eating should not be associated with the regular use of inappropriate compensatory behaviours (e.g., self-induced vomiting; misuse of laxatives, diuretics, or other medications; fasting; or excessive exercise) and not occur exclusively during the course of anorexia nervosa or bulimia nervosa.

The DSM-5 also includes, among the other specified feeding or eating disorders, BED of low frequency and/or limited duration, in which all the criteria for BED are met, except that binge eating is exhibited, on average, less than once a week and/or for less than 3 months. It is worth noting that the DSM-5 diagnostic criteria for BED do not require the presence of obesity or the overvaluation of shape and weight. However, both characteristics are frequently associated with the disorder, as evidenced by clinical samples [4].

Unlike the DSM-5, the International Classification of Diseases, 11th Revision (ICD-11) does not require a large amount of food to be eaten for the definition of binge eating [5]. Indeed, according to the ICD-11, "binge eating is defined as a discrete period of time (e.g., 2 hours) during which the individual experiences a loss of control over their eating behaviour and eats notably more or differently than usual". The decision to adopt broader criteria in the ICD-11 definition of the binge-eating episode, i.e., including both objective and subjective binge eating, was made in order that the diagnosis of BED be more clinically useful, because it is more in line with the lived experience of patients with BED. Indeed, patients with this disorder generally report that loss of control and the perception of overeating are more critical in characterizing the distress experienced around the binge-eating episode than the amount of food consumed [6].

1.2 Epidemiology

No incidence studies on BED have been published. However, it has been widely reported as the most prevalent eating disorder among adults, occurring in both men and women, irrespective of ethnicity or race [7]. Unlike other eating disorders, i.e., anorexia nervosa and bulimia nervosa, where the female-to-male ratio is 9:1, in BED the proportion is more evenly balanced, about 6:4 [8], and its prevalence is comparable across ethnic/racial groups [9].

In the U.S., the 12-month prevalence of BED among adult (age 18 or older) women and men is 1.6 and 0.8%, respectively [1], and does not seem to have increased with the new DSM-5 criteria [10, 11]. The World Health Organization's (WHO) Mental Health Study, which looked at adults in 14 countries across four continents, estimated the median lifetime prevalence of BED as 1.4% (0.8–1.9% interquartile range) [12]. The most recent NESARC-III data (based on the 2012–2013 National Epidemiologic Survey on Alcohol and Related Conditions-III), pertaining to 36,000 U.S. adults, showed a lifetime prevalence in population samples not seeking treatment of 0.85% (men 0.42% and women 1.25%) [9]. However, lifetime prevalence estimates range from less than 1% in several European countries to 4.7% in urbanized areas of Brazil [10].

BED is also the most common eating disorder in adolescence In the U.S. population, it is present in about 1.3% of adolescents [13], and it is more common in those who identify as gay or bisexual, as well as in Native American teenagers and those living in lower-income households [14]. Only 11.9% of adolescents with BED seek clinical care [15], highlighting the importance of prevention and early identification.

1.3 Course

Little information is available on the course of BED, but it has been estimated that it persists for about 16 years on average [9]. It can arise at any age, although in typical cases it develops in late adolescence or young adulthood, generally from 14 to 30 years of age, with a mean age of onset at about 21 years [16]. The first sign is usually binge-eating, often in association with stressful events. Patients generally cycle through prolonged periods of recurrent binge-eating episodes, whose frequency increases during times of stress, and extended interludes free of this behaviour [17]. As binge eating often leads to weight gain, some individuals make several attempts to lose weight without, however, achieving lasting weight loss in the majority of cases [17]. This process is the opposite of what usually occurs in bulimia nervosa, in which the diet usually *precedes* the onset of binge-eating episodes, although in some cases binge eating in BED may begin after a period of strict dieting. That being said, migration from BED to bulimia nervosa or anorexia nervosa is rare.

The main distinction between BED and bulimia nervosa is that, in the former, binge-eating episodes occur in the context of overeating and dysregulated eating, rather than dietary restraint as in the latter. This behaviour explains the disorder's strong association with clinical obesity (see Sect. 4.3.1 and Table 4.4 for the definition).

1.4 Coexistence with Clinical Obesity

Although individuals with BED may present with a BMI in the normal range, it is more frequent in those with clinical obesity. This is explained by the high calorie intake during binge-eating episodes, which, when frequent, tend to result in weight gain that is more or less persistent [17]. Among people seeking treatment for clinical obesity, between 1.4% and 9% meet the DSM diagnostic criteria for BED [18–20], although, in the same population, recurrent binge-eating episodes have been reported in percentages ranging from 9% to 29% [18–20]. In bariatric surgery candidates with a BMI ≥50.0, recurrent binge-eating episodes were reported in up to 50% of cases [21].

For the purposes of comparison, Table 1.1 shows the respective prevalence of the eating disorders diagnosed, via the Eating Disorder Examination interview [22, 23], among 2,810 consecutive patients seeking treatment for clinical obesity at the Department of Eating and Weight Disorders at Villa Garda Hospital, Italy [24]. The cumulative prevalence of BED and BED with low frequency and/or limited duration was 9.5%.

1.5 Other Medical Comorbidities

Most of the physical complications associated with BED appear to be weight-related, and more than 50% of people with BED have at least one comorbid somatic condition. The most frequently diagnosed comorbidities are cardiometabolic diseases such

Table 1.1 Prevalence of eating disorders diagnosed in consecutive treatment-seeking patients with clinical obesity[a]

Eating disorder diagnosis	n.	%
BED	184	6.5
BED with low frequency and/ or limited duration	83	3
Bulimia nervosa	23	0.8
Bulimia nervosa of low frequency and/ or limited duration	57	2
No eating disorder	2,462	87.6
Total	2,810	100

BED binge-eating disorder

[a]Diagnosis made using the Eating Disorder Examination interview [22, 23]

as type 2 diabetes, high blood pressure, hypercholesterolemia, hypertriglyceridemia, and metabolic syndrome [25]. However, one study found that, even after adjusting for BMI, BED was independently associated with elevated blood glucose levels, cardiovascular disease and severe walking limitations, as well as age, sex, schooling, and psychiatric/emotional health indicators [26]. In addition, a longitudinal study with a follow-up of 2.5 years observed that, after adjusting for baseline BMI, BMI change interval, age, and sex, individuals with BED had a higher frequency of newly diagnosed components of metabolic syndrome (dyslipidaemia, arterial hypertension, and type 2 diabetes) [27]. These findings indicate that BED appears to confer a greater risk to cardiometabolic health than clinical obesity alone.

1.6 Psychological Issues

Several psychological problems often coexist with BED. The most common is overvaluation of shape and weight, i.e., judging oneself predominantly or even exclusively on the basis of body shape and weight. This appears to be present in about 50% of individuals with BED [28], who may have more severe overall psychopathology and psychological harm (i.e., depression, low self-esteem and worse quality of life) than those with BED but not overvaluation of shape and weight [29–31], as confirmed by a meta-analysis of 32 studies [32]. In addition, overvaluation of shape and weight appears to be a negative predictor of treatment response to BED [28, 33]. As a consequence, overvaluation of shape and weight has been proposed as a psychopathological marker and specifier of the severity of BED [34, 35].

Other constructs, distinct from but related to the overevaluation of shape and weight, seen in a subgroup of patients with BED are self-criticism, low self-esteem, depressive symptoms [36], and internalized weight stigma (IWB) [37]. The latter involves applying negative weight-based stereotypes to oneself, and engaging in self-blame for one's weight [38]. It is associated with adverse mental health outcomes including depression, anxiety, poor self-esteem and body image, disordered eating, and impaired mental health-related quality of life (HRQoL) [39]. IWB is higher in adults with BED and obesity, as compared to a community sample of adults with obesity alone [40], and in BED it appears to be linked to reduced self-efficacy (i.e., confidence in the ability to control one's eating behaviour in challenging situations) and higher eating disinhibition [41].

Several patients with BED also report general interpersonal difficulties [42], ranging from disputes with family members or significant others to difficulties in developing and maintaining friendships and emotional connections. Specific interpersonal problems include poor flexibility and ineffective interpersonal styles, such as being too dominant or submissive [43].

1.7 Psychiatric Comorbidities

BED often (in up to 90% of cases) coexists with specific psychiatric disorders, particularly major depression; bipolar disorder; anxiety disorders, especially generalized anxiety disorder and panic disorder; post-traumatic stress disorder; and, to a lesser extent, substance and alcohol use disorders and impulse control disorders (e.g., attention-deficit hyperactivity disorder) [9, 16, 25, 44]. The association between BED and psychiatric comorbidities remains even after controlling for body weight [4]. Increased appetite and weight are also included in the diagnostic criteria for atypical forms of major depression and bipolar disorder. In said conditions, increased appetite may or may not be associated with losing control over eating. Only if the latter feature is present in depressive disorder can BED be diagnosed as a coexisting condition [45]. It is important to note that individuals with BED also appear to be at elevated risk of suicide attempts, even after accounting for the presence of other psychiatric disorders and adjusting for sociodemographic factors [46].

1.8 Quality of Life

Individuals with BED are distressed by their eating behaviour and, as stated above, unhappy with the way they look and feel. They often have low self-esteem, which, along with the other features, can impair psychosocial functioning and negatively affect their physical and psychosocial quality of life [47]. This was confirmed by NESARC-III, in which about half of individuals with BED reported interference with normal daily activities [9]. In another survey, 63% of adults with BED reported alterations in school/work functioning, social life, and family life, and nearly 20% reported severe functional impairment [8]. The association of the disorder with clinical obesity and depression further aggravates the physical and mental quality of life, respectively [45]. Poor physical fitness has also been found in individuals with BED [48], which seems to be partly negatively affected by clinical obesity and depression, both often coexistent with this eating disorders [45].

1.9 Differential Diagnosis

1.9.1 Bulimia Nervosa

BED shares recurrent objective binge-eating episodes with bulimia nervosa, but differs from it in four main ways [45]:

1. The recurrent compensatory behaviours seen in bulimia nervosa (self-induced vomiting and/or laxative/diuretics misuse) are not regularly seen in BED.
2. Unlike individuals with bulimia nervosa, those with BED do not show high levels of dietary restraint (i.e., the attempt to restrict eating to change body weight and shape) between binge-eating episodes, although they do report frequent intermittent attempts at weight loss through dysfunctional dieting.
3. The rate of response to treatments is better in individuals with BED than in those with bulimia nervosa.
4. Overvaluation of shape and weight is always present in individuals with bulimia nervosa, but reported in only 50% of individuals with BED.

1.9.2 Night Eating Syndrome

Night eating syndrome is a disorder that is still not well defined, but has three main features [49]: (i) food intake in the evening after dinner or during nocturnal awakenings; (ii) awareness of what one is eating during evening or night-time eating episodes; and (iii) discomfort and impairment resulting from this mode of eating. The disorder usually begins in adolescence and persists continuously into adulthood, although some individuals report longer or shorter periods free of night eating. It affects males and females in equal proportion, and appears to have a hereditary basis. There are four main differences that set night eating syndrome apart from BED [45]:

1. Food intake during night eating episodes is modest (about 300 kcal).
2. Episodes are not generally accompanied by a feeling of loss of control.
3. The motivation to eat is frequently dictated by the fear of being unable to sleep.
4. Night eating episodes occur only in the evening after dinner and/or during nocturnal awakenings.

1.9.3 Binge Eating

Binge eating is not an eating disorder, but rather an eating behaviour. It does not always progress to an eating disorder, although it is a risk factor for BED. Indeed, children who report episodes of loss of control over eating, whether binging objectively or subjectively, have a higher risk of developing BED in adolescence [50].

Furthermore, binge eating occurs in other eating disorders, such as in all the people with bulimia nervosa and many with anorexia nervosa.

1.9.4 Overeating

Overeating, eating more than one wants or has planned, is very common in the general population. It typically occurs during social events and/or meals, and is often associated with positive mood and/or festive occasions (e.g., Christmas lunch). After an overeating episode, people sometimes regret doing so, saying something like, "*I really shouldn't have eaten so much*", but do not experience real distress. This mode of excessive eating is common and is considered normal behaviour, as is frequent snacking (eating small amounts of food) during the day.

Binge-eating episodes, on the other hand, are characterized by the association of eating a large amount of food and feeling a loss of control (i.e., not being able to stop oneself from eating). They are generally followed by disgust, shame, and guilt, but this is quite different from the regret felt after an episode of overeating.

1.10 Treatment

In recent years, several treatments for BED have been proposed and assessed.

1.10.1 Psychological Treatments

The efficacy of cognitive behavioural therapy (CBT) is supported by several systematic reviews and meta-analyses [51], and is recommended as the treatment of choice for BED by the NICE guidelines [52]. Some research has provided support for other specialized psychological treatments for BED, particularly interpersonal psychotherapy (IPT), a form of CBT-based self-help (CBTgsh) [51], and dialectical behavioural therapy (DBT) [7]. In general, psychological treatments result in remission of binge-eating episodes and improvements in the associated eating-disorder and depressive psychopathology in about 50–55% of patients [51]. Although these beneficial effects are maintained at 24 and 48 months [53], these treatments do not generally produce significant weight loss in patients with obesity [54],

1.10.2 Behaviour Weight-Loss Therapy

The challenge of helping BED patients achieve healthy weight loss has been addressed via various strategies. Behaviour weight-loss therapy (BWLT) has been studied as an alternative to CBT for BED because it produces both modest weight loss and remission of binge-eating episodes. For this reason it has also been studied as a sequential intervention to be prescribed after an initial phase of

CBT. Unfortunately, the effects of BWLT on binge-eating episodes are not as well maintained as those seen after CBT, and any weight lost is generally regained [51]. A recent meta-analysis found that individuals with BED lose less weight on BWLT and have a 50% higher treatment abandonment rate than those without BED [55].

1.10.3 Sequential and Combined Treatments

As combining treatments for BED is a relatively new strategy, there is no long-term follow-up data currently available. Nonetheless, in the short term, sequential CBT and BWLT treatment does not appear to produce better results than CBT alone [51], and, in fact, research has not yet demonstrated that any other treatment may be superior to CBT. Other approaches tested to date have combined CBT with medications for weight loss [56], dietary intervention [57], and physical activity programmes [58]. However, these combined strategies provided no appreciable gains in terms of either weight loss or eating-disorder psychopathology improvement, which in fact was significantly reduced with respect to CBT alone. Likewise, a study comparing CBT-E with a multidisciplinary treatment approach integrating CBT-E and weight management methods [59], found that the latter produced a lower weight loss than that habitually achieved by BWLT. Specifically, only 25% of participants had achieved a >5% weight loss at 12 months, likely due to the weight management component being insufficient [59].

1.10.4 Medications

Several medications have been tested as treatments for BED, including antidepressants (selective serotonin-reuptake inhibitors, serotonin, norepinephrine reuptake inhibitors, and bupropion), anticonvulsants (topiramate), weight-loss agents (sibutramine), and drugs prescribed for the treatment of substance-use disorders (naltrexone) [51, 60]. Although some antidepressants can reduce the frequency of binge-eating episodes, they are often associated with weight gain. Topiramate, although shown to reduce both the frequency of binge-eating episodes and weight, is not recommended because it may damage cognitive function.

In 2015, the Food and Drug Administration (FDA) approved lisdexamfetamine for the treatment of BED. This approval was granted because it was shown to be superior to a placebo in reducing binge-eating episodes and associated obsessive–compulsive symptoms in three randomized controlled trials (remission of binge-eating episodes after 12 weeks: 36–50% LDX vs. 13–21% placebo) [61]. It also appears to reduce the relapse rate as compared to placebo at 24 weeks' follow-up (32.1% vs. 3.7%) in patients who responded (classed as those with $\leq$1 binge-eating episode per day over the last 4 weeks) during a 12-week open-label treatment phase [62]. It should be noted, however, that LDX is not indicated for weight loss or the treatment of obesity, and is unavailable in Europe. Not only does it have a high potential for abuse/addiction, but also a recent study found that long-term exposure to this medication is associated with an increased risk of cardiovascular disease [63].

The latest-generation medications for clinical obesity have also been tested as treatments for BED in some studies. However, neither naltrexone/bupropion [64] nor liraglutide [65] showed any greater efficacy in reducing binge eating than placebo, despite effectively reducing patients' weight. However, the liraglutide study had a significant flaw, namely erroneous dispensing of drugs in pharmacies, and further research into the use of GLP-1 agonists as treatments of BED associated with obesity is therefore warranted.

1.10.5 Clinical Obesity Management in BED

While there are effective options for both clinical obesity and BED, there is as yet none available for the two in concomitance. Hence, there is a pressing need to develop a treatment that simultaneously effects remission of binge-eating and the associated psychopathology, and enables good management of clinical obesity (see Chap. 4) and its complications. Such a treatment would need to bring about clinically significant weight loss [54] without the adverse effects that often accompany drugs proposed for BED. This objective is paramount because the data consistently indicates that even patients who manage to abstain from binge-eating episodes maintain their weight at the end of treatment, including any modest weight gain they have achieved during its course [51]. With this in mind, we set about developing the new, integrated, treatment described in the following chapters of this book. It explicitly aims to achieve two fundamental goals in patients with BED, namely remission of binge-eating episodes and healthy weight loss (if indicated).

References

1. American Psychiatric Association. Diagnostic and statistical manual of mental disorders, (DSM-5). Arlington: American Psychiatric Publishing; 2013.
2. Engel SG, Kahler KA, Lystad CM, Crosby RD, Simonich HK, Wonderlich SA, et al. Eating behavior in obese BED, obese non-BED, and non-obese control participants: a naturalistic study. Behav Res Ther. 2009;47(10):897–900. https://doi.org/10.1016/j.brat.2009.06.018.
3. Fairburn CG, Wilson GT. In Binge eating: definition and classification. In Fairburn CG, Wilson GT, editors. Binge eating: nature, assessment, and treatment. New York: Guilford Press; 1993. p. 3–14
4. Devlin MJ. Binge eating disorder. In: Brownell KD, Walsh BT, editors. Eating disorders and obesity. New York: Guilford Press; 2017. p. 192–7.
5. World Health Organization: International classification of diseases for mortality and morbidity statistics (11th Revision). https://icd.who.int/browse11/l-m/en (2018). Accessed.
6. Hay P. Current approach to eating disorders: a clinical update. Intern Med J. 2020;50(1):24–9. https://doi.org/10.1111/imj.14691.
7. Grilo CM, Juarascio A. Binge-eating disorder interventions: review, current status, and implications. Curr Obes Rep. 2023; https://doi.org/10.1007/s13679-023-00517-0.

8. Hudson JI, Hiripi E, Pope HG Jr, Kessler RC. The prevalence and correlates of eating disorders in the National Comorbidity Survey Replication. Biol Psychiatry. 2007;61(3):348–58. https://doi.org/10.1016/j.biopsych.2006.03.040.
9. Udo T, Grilo CM. Prevalence and correlates of DSM-5-defined eating disorders in a nationally representative sample of U.S. adults. Biol Psychiatry. 2018;84(5):345–54. https://doi.org/10.1016/j.biopsych.2018.03.014.
10. Smink FR, van Hoeken D, Hoek HW. Epidemiology, course, and outcome of eating disorders. Curr Opin Psychiatry. 2013;26(6):543–8. https://doi.org/10.1097/YCO.0b013e328365a24f.
11. Trace SE, Thornton LM, Root TL, Mazzeo SE, Lichtenstein P, Pedersen NL, et al. Effects of reducing the frequency and duration criteria for binge eating on lifetime prevalence of bulimia nervosa and binge eating disorder: implications for DSM-5. Int J Eat Disord. 2012;45(4):531–6. https://doi.org/10.1002/eat.20955.
12. Kessler RC, Berglund PA, Chiu WT, Deitz AC, Hudson JI, Shahly V, et al. The prevalence and correlates of binge eating disorder in the World Health Organization World Mental Health Surveys. Biol Psychiatry. 2013;73(9):904–14. https://doi.org/10.1016/j.biopsych.2012.11.020.
13. Kjeldbjerg ML, Clausen L. Prevalence of binge-eating disorder among children and adolescents: a systematic review and meta-analysis. Eur Child Adolesc Psychiatry. 2023;32(4):549–74. https://doi.org/10.1007/s00787-021-01850-2.
14. Nagata JM, Smith-Russack Z, Paul A, Saldana GA, Shao IY, Al-Shoaibi AAA, et al. The social epidemiology of binge-eating disorder and behaviors in early adolescents. J Eat Disord. 2023;11(1):182. https://doi.org/10.1186/s40337-023-00904-x.
15. Swanson SA, Crow SJ, Le Grange D, Swendsen J, Merikangas KR. Prevalence and correlates of eating disorders in adolescents. Results from the national comorbidity survey replication adolescent supplement. Arch Gen Psychiatry. 2011;68(7):714–23. https://doi.org/10.1001/archgenpsychiatry.2011.22.
16. Citrome L. Binge-eating disorder and comorbid conditions: differential diagnosis and implications for treatment. J Clin Psychiatry. 2017;78(Suppl 1):9–13. https://doi.org/10.4088/JCP.sh16003su1c.02.
17. Fairburn CG. Overcoming binge eating. 2nd ed. New York: Guilford Press; 2013.
18. Gorin AA, Niemeier HM, Hogan P, Coday M, Davis C, DiLillo VG, et al. Binge eating and weight loss outcomes in overweight and obese individuals with type 2 diabetes: results from the Look AHEAD trial. Arch Gen Psychiatry. 2008;65(12):1447–55. https://doi.org/10.1001/archpsyc.65.12.1447.
19. Ricca V, Mannucci E, Moretti S, Di Bernardo M, Zucchi T, Cabras PL, et al. Screening for binge eating disorder in obese outpatients. Compr Psychiatry. 2000;41(2):111–5. https://doi.org/10.1016/s0010-440x(00)90143-3.
20. Allison KC, Crow SJ, Reeves RR, West DS, Foreyt JP, Dilillo VG, et al. Binge eating disorder and night eating syndrome in adults with type 2 diabetes. Obesity (Silver Spring, Md). 2007;15(5):1287–93. https://doi.org/10.1038/oby.2007.150.
21. Vinai P, Da Ros A, Speciale M, Gentile N, Tagliabue A, Vinai P, et al. Psychopathological characteristics of patients seeking for bariatric surgery, either affected or not by binge eating disorder following the criteria of the DSM IV TR and of the DSM 5. Eat Behav. 2015;16:1–4. https://doi.org/10.1016/j.eatbeh.2014.10.004.
22. Calugi S, Ricca V, Castellini G, Lo Sauro C, Ruocco A, Chignola E, et al. The Eating Disorder Examination: reliability and validity of the Italian version. Eat Weight Disord. 2015;20(4):505–11. https://doi.org/10.1007/s40519-015-0191-2.
23. Fairburn CG, Cooper Z, O'Connor M. Eating disorder examination. In: Fairburn CG, editor. Cognitive behavior therapy and eating disorders. New York: Guilford Press; 2008. p. 265–308.
24. Dalle Grave R. Obesity and eating disorders: an interactive and complex coexistence. IJEDO. 2023:5. https://doi.org/10.32044/ijedo.2023.04.
25. Udo T, Grilo CM. Psychiatric and medical correlates of DSM-5 eating disorders in a nationally representative sample of adults in the United States. Int J Eat Disord. 2019;52(1):42–50. https://doi.org/10.1002/eat.23004.

26. Mitchell JE, King WC, Pories W, Wolfe B, Flum DR, Spaniolas K, et al. Binge eating disorder and medical comorbidities in bariatric surgery candidates. Int J Eat Disord. 2015;48(5):471–6. https://doi.org/10.1002/eat.22389.
27. Hudson JI, Lalonde JK, Coit CE, Tsuang MT, McElroy SL, Crow SJ, et al. Longitudinal study of the diagnosis of components of the metabolic syndrome in individuals with binge-eating disorder. Am J Clin Nutr. 2010;91(6):1568–73. https://doi.org/10.3945/ajcn.2010.29203.
28. Grilo CM. Why no cognitive body image feature such as overvaluation of shape/weight in the binge eating disorder diagnosis? Int J Eat Disord. 2013;46(3):208–11. https://doi.org/10.1002/eat.22082.
29. Grilo CM, Hrabosky JI, White MA, Allison KC, Stunkard AJ, Masheb RM. Overvaluation of shape and weight in binge eating disorder and overweight controls: refinement of a diagnostic construct. J Abnorm Psychol. 2008;117(2):414–9. https://doi.org/10.1037/0021-843x.117.2.414.
30. Hrabosky JI, Masheb RM, White MA, Grilo CM. Overvaluation of shape and weight in binge eating disorder. J Consult Clin Psychol. 2007;75(1):175–80. https://doi.org/10.1037/0022-006x.75.1.175.
31. Mond JM, Hay PJ, Rodgers B, Owen C. Recurrent binge eating with and without the "undue influence of weight or shape on self-evaluation": implications for the diagnosis of binge eating disorder. Behav Res Ther. 2007;45(5):929–38. https://doi.org/10.1016/j.brat.2006.08.011.
32. Linardon J. Correlates of the over-evaluation of weight and shape in binge eating disorder and mixed eating disorder samples: a meta-analytic review. Eat Disord. 2017;25(3):183–98. https://doi.org/10.1080/10640266.2016.1260374.
33. Masheb RM, Grilo CM. Prognostic significance of two sub-categorization methods for the treatment of binge eating disorder: negative affect and overvaluation predict, but do not moderate, specific outcomes. Behav Res Ther. 2008;46(4):428–37. https://doi.org/10.1016/j.brat.2008.01.004.
34. Grilo CM, White MA, Gueorguieva R, Wilson GT, Masheb RM. Predictive significance of the overvaluation of shape/weight in obese patients with binge eating disorder: findings from a randomized controlled trial with 12-month follow-up. Psychol Med. 2013;43(6):1335–44. https://doi.org/10.1017/s0033291712002097.
35. Grilo CM, Ivezaj V, White MA. Evaluation of the DSM-5 severity indicator for binge eating disorder in a community sample. Behav Res Ther. 2015;66:72–6. https://doi.org/10.1016/j.brat.2015.01.004.
36. Dunkley DM, Grilo CM. Self-criticism, low self-esteem, depressive symptoms, and over-evaluation of shape and weight in binge eating disorder patients. Behav Res Ther. 2007;45(1):139–49. https://doi.org/10.1016/j.brat.2006.01.017.
37. Wang SB, Lydecker JA, Grilo CM. Rumination in patients with binge-eating disorder and obesity: associations with eating-disorder psychopathology and weight-bias internalization. Eur Eat Disord Rev. 2017;25(2):98–103. https://doi.org/10.1002/erv.2499.
38. Pearl RL, Puhl RM. Measuring internalized weight attitudes across body weight categories: validation of the modified weight bias internalization scale. Body Image. 2014;11(1):89–92. https://doi.org/10.1016/j.bodyim.2013.09.005.
39. Pearl RL, Puhl RM. Weight bias internalization and health: a systematic review. Obes Rev. 2018;19(8):1141–63. https://doi.org/10.1111/obr.12701.
40. Durso LE, Latner JD, White MA, Masheb RM, Blomquist KK, Morgan PT, et al. Internalized weight bias in obese patients with binge eating disorder: associations with eating disturbances and psychological functioning. Int J Eat Disord. 2012;45(3):423–7. https://doi.org/10.1002/eat.20933.
41. Groshon LC, Pearl RL. Longitudinal associations of binge eating with internalized weight stigma and eating self-efficacy. Eat Behav. 2023;50:101785. https://doi.org/10.1016/j.eatbeh.2023.101785.
42. Blomquist KK, Ansell EB, White MA, Masheb RM, Grilo CM. Interpersonal problems and developmental trajectories of binge eating disorder. Compr Psychiatry. 2012;53(8):1088–95. https://doi.org/10.1016/j.comppsych.2012.05.003.
43. Wilfley DE, Eichen DM. Intrepersonal psychotherapy. In: Brownell KD, Walsh BT, editors. Eating disorders and obesity. New York: Guilford Press; 2017. p. 290–5.

44. Grilo CM, Udo T. Posttraumatic stress disorder and binge-eating disorder: further context and additional findings from a nationally representative sample of adults in the united states. J Clin Psychiatry. 2020;81(2) https://doi.org/10.4088/JCP.19lr13157.
45. Dalle Grave R. Disturbo da alimentazione incontrollata. Che cos'è e come affrontarlo. Verona: Positive Press; 2014.
46. Udo T, Bitley S, Grilo CM. Suicide attempts in US adults with lifetime DSM-5 eating disorders. BMC Med. 2019;17(1):120. https://doi.org/10.1186/s12916-019-1352-3.
47. Agh T, Kovacs G, Pawaskar M, Supina D, Inotai A, Voko Z. Epidemiology, health-related quality of life and economic burden of binge eating disorder: a systematic literature review. Eat Weight Disord. 2015;20(1):1–12. https://doi.org/10.1007/s40519-014-0173-9.
48. Mathisen TF, Rosenvinge JH, Friborg O, Pettersen G, Stensrud T, Hansen BH, et al. Body composition and physical fitness in women with bulimia nervosa or binge-eating disorder. Int J Eat Disord. 2018;51(4):331–42. https://doi.org/10.1002/eat.22841.
49. O'Reardon JP, Peshek A, Allison KC. Night eating syndrome: diagnosis, epidemiology and management. CNS Drugs. 2005;19(12):997–1008. https://doi.org/10.2165/00023210-200519120-00003.
50. Hilbert A, Brauhardt A. Childhood loss of control eating over five-year follow-up. Int J Eat Disord. 2014;47(7):758–61. https://doi.org/10.1002/eat.22312.
51. Hilbert A, Petroff D, Herpertz S, Pietrowsky R, Tuschen-Caffier B, Vocks S, et al. Meta-analysis of the efficacy of psychological and medical treatments for binge-eating disorder. J Consult Clin Psychol. 2019;87(1):91–105. https://doi.org/10.1037/ccp0000358.
52. National Guideline Alliance. Eating disorders: recognition and treatment. London: National Institute for Health and Care Excellence (UK); 2017 May. (NICE Guideline, No. 69.). London: 2017.
53. Hilbert A, Bishop ME, Stein RI, Tanofsky-Kraff M, Swenson AK, Welch RR, et al. Long-term efficacy of psychological treatments for binge eating disorder. Br J Psychiatry. 2012;200(3):232–7. https://doi.org/10.1192/bjp.bp.110.089664.
54. Cooper Z, Calugi S, Dalle GR. Controlling binge eating and weight: a treatment for binge eating disorder worth researching? Eat Weight Disord. 2019;25(4):1105–9. https://doi.org/10.1007/s40519-019-00734-4.
55. Forman EM, Evans BC, Berry MP, Lampe EW, Chwyl C, Zhang F. Behavioral weight loss outcomes in individuals with binge-eating disorder: a meta-analysis. Obesity. 2023;31(8):1981–95. https://doi.org/10.1002/oby.23790.
56. Grilo CM, Masheb RM, Salant SL. Cognitive behavioral therapy guided self-help and orlistat for the treatment of binge eating disorder: a randomized, double-blind, placebo-controlled trial. Biol Psychiatry. 2005;57(10):1193–201. https://doi.org/10.1016/j.biopsych.2005.03.001.
57. Masheb RM, Grilo CM, Rolls BJ. A randomized controlled trial for obesity and binge eating disorder: low-energy-density dietary counseling and cognitive-behavioral therapy. Behav Res Ther. 2011;49(12):821–9. https://doi.org/10.1016/j.brat.2011.09.006.
58. Blanchet C, Mathieu ME, St-Laurent A, Fecteau S, St-Amour N, Drapeau V. A systematic review of physical activity interventions in individuals with binge eating disorders. Curr Obes Rep. 2018;7(1):76–88. https://doi.org/10.1007/s13679-018-0295-x.
59. Palavras MA, Hay P, Mannan H, da Luz FQ, Sainsbury A, Touyz S, et al. Integrated weight loss and cognitive behavioural therapy (CBT) for the treatment of recurrent binge eating and high body mass index: a randomized controlled trial. Eat Weight Disord. 2021;26(1):249–62. https://doi.org/10.1007/s40519-020-00846-2.
60. Citrome L. Binge eating disorder revisited: what's new, what's different, what's next—Addendum. CNS Spectr. 2019;24(S1):82. https://doi.org/10.1017/S1092852919001366.
61. Citrome L. Lisdexamfetamine for binge eating disorder in adults: a systematic review of the efficacy and safety profile for this newly approved indication—what is the number needed to treat, number needed to harm and likelihood to be helped or harmed? Int J Clin Pract. 2015;69(4):410–21. https://doi.org/10.1111/ijcp.12639.

62. Hudson JI, McElroy SL, Ferreira-Cornwell MC, Radewonuk J, Gasior M. Efficacy of lisdexamfetamine in adults with moderate to severe binge-eating disorder: a randomized clinical trial. JAMA Psychiatry. 2017;74(9):903–10. https://doi.org/10.1001/jamapsychiatry.2017.1889.
63. Zhang L, Li L, Andell P, Garcia-Argibay M, Quinn PD, D'Onofrio BM, et al. Attention-deficit/hyperactivity disorder medications and long-term risk of cardiovascular diseases. JAMA Psychiatry. 2023; https://doi.org/10.1001/jamapsychiatry.2023.4294.
64. Grilo CM, Lydecker JA, Jastreboff AM, Pittman B, McKee SA. Naltrexone/bupropion for binge-eating disorder: a randomized, double-blind, placebo-controlled trial. Obesity. 2023; https://doi.org/10.1002/oby.23898.
65. Allison KC, Chao AM, Bruzas MB, McCuen-Wurst C, Jones E, McAllister C, et al. A pilot randomized controlled trial of liraglutide 3.0 mg for binge eating disorder. Obes Sci Pract. 2023;9(2):127–36. https://doi.org/10.1002/osp4.619.

Cognitive Behaviour Theory

2

Abstract

The cognitive behaviour theory of binge-eating disorder (BED) integrates established transdiagnostic mechanisms that maintain binge-eating episodes with the cognitive and behavioural factors that play a role in the perpetuation of clinical obesity. The model hypothesizes that events triggering mood changes, overvaluation of shape and weight, and dysfunctional dieting contribute to the continuance of binge-eating episodes, mirroring their role in other eating disorders. The model is innovative in that it acknowledges the need to address dysregulated eating and overeating between binge-eating episodes, as well as sedentary lifestyle, unrealistic weight-loss goals and associated primary goals (see below), and internalized weight stigma.

The model integrates the known mechanisms behind binge-eating episodes that have previously been incorporated into the transdiagnostic theory and treatment of eating disorders (Fig. 2.1) [1, 2]. It suggests that of overvaluation of shape and weight, events and associated mood changes, and dysfunctional dieting contribute to maintaining binge-eating episodes in the same way that they operate in other eating disorders. The model also encompasses behavioural factors that contribute to the onset and persistence of clinical obesity (i.e., when an individual's physical health and or psychosocial functioning is significantly impaired due to obesity). This is due to the fact that generally unhealthy eating patterns as well as binge-eating episodes, in addition to sedentary lifestyle, unrealistic weight-loss and other (primary) goals [3], and internalized weight stigma, if present, represent obstacles to the long-term recovery of patients with BED and clinical obesity. While that not all of the above maintenance factors operate in all cases of BED, all cases of BED feature a combination thereof.

R. Dalle Grave et al., *Cognitive Behavior Therapy for Binge Eating Disorder*, https://doi.org/10.1007/978-3-031-71456-6_2

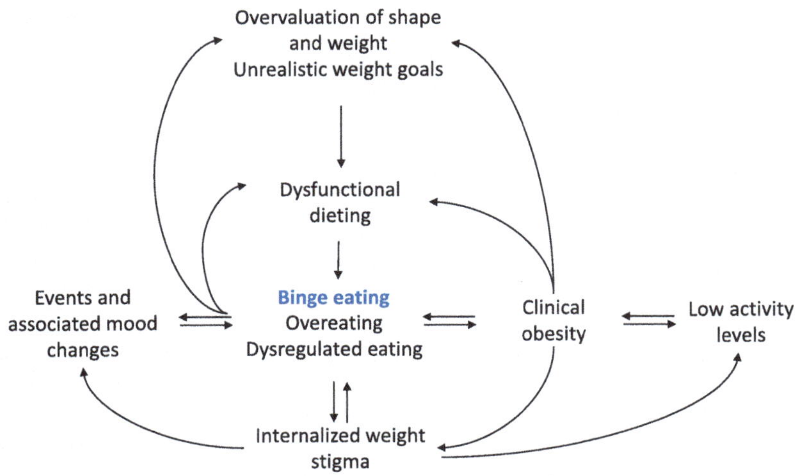

Fig. 2.1 The main mechanisms that maintain binge eating according to cognitive behavioural theory

2.1 Events and Associated Mood Changes

Life events and associated mood changes often trigger and maintain (i.e., reinforce) binge-eating episodes in people with BED [4]. The association between life events, emotional changes, and binge-eating episodes can be explained by the following observations [1]:

- Food may be used to distract oneself from adverse events and problems.
- Food may help mitigate emotional states.
- Food can be a means of self-gratification.

However, after an initial attenuation of the negative emotional state, a binge-eating episode often leads to feelings of guilt, anxiety, and depression, which can, in turn, trigger a further binge-eating episode.

A subgroup of people with BED report a co-existing problem known as "mood intolerance". This expression is used to describe the experience of individuals who are exceptionally sensitive to emotions, have frequent negative emotions (e.g., anger, anxiety), and find it difficult to tolerate and manage them. Those who suffer from this problem adopt dysfunctional mood-modulating behaviours, such as taking psychoactive substances (alcohol or tranquilizers) or binge eating, which reduce awareness of the emotional state (and associated thoughts). However, such unhealthy coping strategies take a significant toll on an individual's emotional, interpersonal, and physical well-being [1].

2.2 Overvaluation of Shape and Weight

A person is described as having overvaluation of shape and weight when they judge their self-worth predominantly, and in some cases exclusively, in terms of their body shape, weight, and their ability to control them [1]. As described in Chap. 1, this is a feature present in about 50% of people with BED [5]. It must be distinguished from body dissatisfaction, a term used when a person does not like their physical appearance [6]. Indeed, body dissatisfaction is widespread in the general population and does not necessarily represent a clinical issue. Overvaluation of shape and weight, on the other hand, marginalizes other areas of life, largely reducing an individual's sphere of interests to their own body. This inevitably lessens their commitment to the major life domains (e.g., school, social relationships, and work) that normally contribute to the development of a functional, stable, and articulated self-evaluation system (Fig. 2.2).

Typically, overvaluation of shape and weight is expressed through frequent body checking (e.g., frequent weighing, scrutiny of body parts, measuring body circumferences, grasping folds of subcutaneous fat, and comparing one's body with that of others), avoidance of weighing oneself and exposing one's body shape, and adopting a strict diet or other extreme weight-control behaviours. In BED, the binge-eating episodes are interspersed with intermittent dysfunctional dieting and/or other unhealthy behaviours in the attempt to lose weight, which in turn make binge eating more likely through the mechanisms described below. Being associated with a greater frequency of binge-eating episodes and more severe psychological distress and psychosocial harm, the overvaluation of shape and weight is considered a specifier of BED severity [5, 7]. It is also a predictor of relapse and heightened eating-disorder psychopathology and depression scores 1 year later in patients who achieved abstinence from binge eating via behaviour therapy [8].

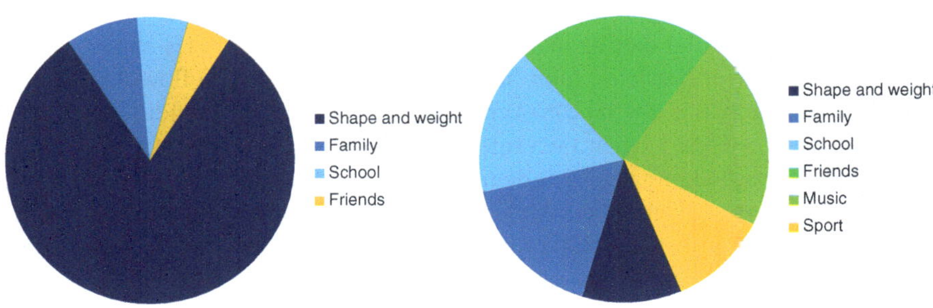

Fig. 2.2 Representative "self-worth" pie chart of a person with (on the left) and without (on the right) an eating disorder. (Note: the size of the slice corresponds to the relative degree of importance attributed to each domain in self-evaluation)

2.3 Unrealistic Weight Goals and Primary Goals

Research data indicate that genetic factors determine 40–70% of interindividual BMI variability [9]. For this reason, a person may only be able to partially modify their body weight. Currently, there are no treatments (except for bariatric surgery and new weight loss drugs) that result in an average long-term weight loss of more than 5–10% of the initial body weight, which nevertheless has a positive effect on quality of life and reduces the main medical complications associated with clinical obesity [10], including cardiovascular mortality [11].

However, people seeking to lose weight often have unrealistic expectations of how much weight they will be able to lose. Studies carried out in Italy indicate that many people who start weight-loss treatment want to lose more than 5–10% of their starting weight (on average, they have a weight-loss goal of 32%) [12]. In addition, they may be harbouring other, "primary" goals that are not necessarily achievable through weight loss, such as improving interpersonal relationships and/or self-confidence, or finding a partner or a new job.

There seems to be a link between unrealistic weight goals and primary goals and treatment discontinuation [13, 14]. They are also associated with an individual's lack of commitment to maintaining the weight lost, a result that they deem to be unsatisfactory if they still adhere to their initial, unachievable expectations [15]. In addition, unrealistic weight goals often prompt people with BED to alternate between binging and extreme weight-control behaviours, one fuelling the other via the mechanisms described below.

2.4 Dysfunctional Dieting

Some people with BED, particularly those who overvalue shape and/or have unrealistic weight goals, attempt to control their weight and change their body shape by intermittently adopting dysfunctional diets characterized by extreme, rigid dietary rules [3]. This pattern of dieting makes further binge-eating episodes almost inevitable (Fig. 2.1), as the stricter, more numerous and difficult to follow the dietary rule, the more likely it is it will be broken. When this occurs, an individual interprets their inability to adhere to their own rules as evidence of their lack of self-control, rather than acknowledging that their dietary rules are too strict and/or extreme. This interpretation ("all-or-nothing thinking") favours the temporary abandonment of a person's efforts to curb their calorie intake, leading them to exchange their weight-control efforts for another binge-eating episode [1].

2.5 Binge Eating

During the binge-eating episode, preference is given to foods that are high in carbohydrates or fats, do not require too much preparation, and are easy to chew (e.g., sweets, ice cream, bread, cakes, chocolate) [16]. However, if there are no sweets or carbohydrates to hand, any food will do. In fact, some eat only foods that they consider healthy (i.e., fruits and vegetables), while others simply increase their portion sizes [16]. Studies have shown that there is no physical dependence on carbohydrates: what characterizes binge-eating episodes is not the quality but the amount of food consumed [16]—typically between 1,000 and 2,000 calories per episode. This high-calorie intake explains why, when binge-eating episodes are frequent, people with BED tend to gain weight and keep it on (Fig. 2.1).

2.6 Overeating and Dysregulated Eating

Between binge-eating episodes, people with BED often overeat, and their eating tends to be dysregulated and characterized by a lack of flexible moderation in food intake. Dysregulated eating behaviours may include skipping meals (e.g., breakfast), frequently snacking or grazing between meals, or eating oversized portions and "junk" foods that are high in calories, saturated fat, sugar, and/or salt (e.g., hamburgers, hot dogs, fried chicken, French fries, sugary drinks, processed desserts, pizza) [17]. In many cases this combination of overconsumption and dysregulated eating leads to an excessive daily intake of calories sufficient to promote the onset and/or maintenance of clinical obesity. It also reinforces a susceptible individual's overvaluation of shape and weight and unrealistic weight goals, leading to bouts of dysfunctional dieting followed by binge-eating episodes (Fig. 2.1).

2.7 Clinical Obesity

Overeating, dysregulated eating without the regular use of compensatory behaviours, and binge eating itself explain why clinical obesity (see Sect. 4.3.1 and Table 4.4 for the definition) is common in people with BED [18–20]. However, genetic factors, obesity, and more exposure to negative comments about shape, weight, and eating in childhood have been shown to increase the risk of BED onset [21]. As shown in Fig. 2.1, clinical obesity increases the risk of developing internalized weight stigma, and fuels the overvaluation of shape and weight, unrealistic weight goals, and intermittent adoption of dysfunctional dieting, dysregulated eating, and overeating (in part also due to some genetic mechanisms implicated in the development of obesity [22]), as well as the binge-eating episodes themselves.

2.8 Sedentary Lifestyle

A large subgroup of people with BED and clinical obesity do very little physical activity during the course of their day. Their energy expenditure is consequently low, and can contribute to the development and maintenance of clinical obesity, which in turn makes it more difficult and less enjoyable to exercise [23] (Fig. 2.1).

2.9 Internalized Weight Stigma

Weight bias is a term used to define negative attitudes towards people perceived to have higher body weight. These irrational attitudes are manifested in stereotypes and/or prejudices towards such people, who are perceived to be weak and/or lazy, unintelligent, unattractive, and lacking willpower and self-discipline. At the root of these attitudes is a moral judgement blaming people with higher body weight for being responsible for their own condition [24]. Such negative stereotypes are rarely challenged in Western society, which in fact promotes the development of *weight stigma*, i.e., societal devaluation or discrediting due to weight [24], on multiple levels [25], namely (i) structural (media, laws & policies); (ii) interpersonal (teasing/bullying, body shaming, discrimination); and (iii) intrapersonal (anticipation, internalization). Widespread weight stigma means that people with higher weight are often marginalized and excluded, leading to inequalities and distress. Both men and women are vulnerable to weight discrimination. However, women, in particular those who are middle-aged or have lower levels of education, experience a higher rate of weight stigmatization than men, even at lower levels of overweight [26].

Internalized weight stigma occurs when individuals apply society's negative weight stereotypes to themselves. These generate negative beliefs about themselves due to their perception of having a large body and being inferior to those who are able to control their weight, resulting in thoughts like *I'm so lazy, I have no will-power, I hate myself for not having any self-control, I'm a failure,* and *I am ugly and disgusting*. Internalized weight stigma can be assessed via the Weight-Bias Internalization Scale (WBIS: 10 or 11 items, each scored 1–7 then averaged) [27] and/or the Weight Self-Stigma Questionnaire (WSSQ: 12 items, each scored 1–5 then added together) [28].

Internalized weight stigma extends beyond body dissatisfaction because of the associated overvaluation of shape and weight. Indeed, individuals who have high internalized weight stigma scores view themselves as a failure on the whole merely because of their weight [29]. Women report a higher level of weight bias internalization than men, and younger individuals have more internalized weight bias than older ones [30]. In women, there is a correlation between a higher BMI and a higher level of internalized stigma [31]. A recent study, on 13,996 adults seeking treatment for obesity in six countries [32], found that, after controlling for participant characteristics and weight stigma experiences, WBIS-M scores were associated with more significant weight gain over the preceding year. Participants with higher WBIS-M scores also reported poorer mental and physical quality of life, lower self-efficacy in eating control and physical activity, more frequent use of food as a coping strategy, greater avoidance of gym attendance, worse body image, and higher perceived stress. Recent research has also found an association between internalized weight stigma and metabolic syndrome [33], unhealthy behaviours [34], low self-efficacy [35], more severe eating-disorder psychopathology [36], and binge eating [37].

People with internalized weight stigma often manage their negative emotions through binge-eating episodes and/or overeating, have little pleasure in doing physical activity and sports, and with a greater tendency to avoid them (Fig. 2.1). At the same time, their low self-efficacy (i.e., an individual's belief in their capacity to put into practice behaviours necessary to achieve specific performance goals [38]) can hamper their attempts to control their eating and weight, and even lead to their avoiding treatment due to fear of failure.

References

1. Fairburn CG. Cognitive behavior therapy and eating disorders. New York: Guilford Press; 2008.
2. Fairburn CG, Cooper Z, Shafran R. Cognitive behaviour therapy for eating disorders: a "transdiagnostic" theory and treatment. Behav Res Ther. 2003;41(5):509–28. https://doi.org/10.1016/s0005-7967(02)00088-8.
3. Cooper Z, Calugi S, Dalle GR. Controlling binge eating and weight a treatment for binge eating disorder worth researching? Eat Weight Disord. 2019;25(4):1105–9. https://doi.org/10.1007/s40519-019-00734-4.
4. Nicholls W, Devonport TJ, Blake M. The association between emotions and eating behaviour in an obese population with binge eating disorder. Obes Rev. 2016;17(1):30–42. https://doi.org/10.1111/obr.12329.
5. Grilo CM, White MA, Gueorguieva R, Wilson GT, Masheb RM. Predictive significance of the overvaluation of shape/weight in obese patients with binge eating disorder: findings from a randomized controlled trial with 12-month follow-up. Psychol Med. 2013;43(6):1335–44. https://doi.org/10.1017/s0033291712002097.
6. Dalle Grave R, Calugi S. Transdiagnostic cognitive behavioural theory and treatment of body image disturbance in eating disorders: a guide to assessment, treatment, and prevention. In: Cuzzolaro M, Fassino S, editors. Body image, eating, and weight. Cham: Springer; 2018. p. 309–21.
7. Grilo CM, Ivezaj V, White MA. Evaluation of the DSM-5 severity indicator for binge eating disorder in a community sample. Behav Res Ther. 2015;66:72–6. https://doi.org/10.1016/j.brat.2015.01.004.
8. Grilo CM, Ivezaj V, Gueorguieva R. Overvaluation of shape/weight at posttreatment predicts relapse at 12-month follow-up after successful behaviorally-based treatment of binge-eating disorder. Int J Eat Disord. 2024; https://doi.org/10.1002/eat.24141.
9. Locke AE, Kahali B, Berndt SI, Justice AE, Pers TH, Day FR, et al. Genetic studies of body mass index yield new insights for obesity biology. Nature. 2015;518(7538):197–206. https://doi.org/10.1038/nature14177.
10. Jensen MD, Ryan DH, Apovian CM, Ard JD, Comuzzie AG, Donato KA, et al. AHA/ACC/TOS guideline for the management of overweight and obesity in adults: a report of the American College of Cardiology/American Heart Association Task Force on Practice Guidelines and The Obesity Society. J Am Coll Cardiol. 2013;63(25 Pt B):2985–3023. https://doi.org/10.1016/j.jacc.2013.11.004.
11. Gregg EW, Jakicic JM, Blackburn G, Bloomquist P, Bray GA, Clark JM, et al. Association of the magnitude of weight loss and changes in physical fitness with long-term cardiovascular disease outcomes in overweight or obese people with type 2 diabetes: a post-hoc analysis of the Look AHEAD randomised clinical trial. Lancet Diabetes Endocrinol. 2016;4(11):913–21. https://doi.org/10.1016/s2213-8587(16)30162-0.
12. Dalle Grave R, Calugi S, Magri F, Cuzzolaro M, Dall'aglio E, Lucchin L, et al. Weight loss expectations in obese patients seeking treatment at medical centers. Obes Res. 2004;12(12):2005–12. https://doi.org/10.1038/oby.2004.251.
13. Dalle Grave R, Calugi S, Molinari E, Petroni ML, Bondi M, Compare A, et al. Weight loss expectations in obese patients and treatment attrition: an observational multicenter study. Obes Res. 2005;13(11):1961–9. https://doi.org/10.1038/oby.2005.241.

14. Dalle Grave R, Calugi S, Compare A, El Ghoch M, Petroni ML, Tomasi F, et al. Weight loss expectations and attrition in treatment-seeking obese women. Obes Facts. 2015;8(5):311–8. https://doi.org/10.1159/000441366.
15. Calugi S, Marchesini G, El Ghoch M, Gavasso I, Dalle GR. The association between weight maintenance and session-by-session diet adherence, weight loss and weight-loss satisfaction. Eat Weight Disord. 2020;25(1):127–33. https://doi.org/10.1007/s40519-018-0528-8.
16. Fairburn CG. Overcoming binge eating. 2nd ed. New York: Guilford Press; 2013.
17. Elran-Barak R, Sztainer M, Goldschmidt AB, Crow SJ, Peterson CB, Hill LL, et al. Dietary restriction behaviors and binge eating in anorexia nervosa, bulimia nervosa and binge eating disorder: trans-diagnostic examination of the restraint model. Eat Behav. 2015;18:192–6. https://doi.org/10.1016/j.eatbeh.2015.05.012.
18. Gorin AA, Niemeier HM, Hogan P, Coday M, Davis C, DiLillo VG, et al. Binge eating and weight loss outcomes in overweight and obese individuals with type 2 diabetes: results from the Look AHEAD trial. Arch Gen Psychiatry. 2008;65(12):1447–55. https://doi.org/10.1001/archpsyc.65.12.1447.
19. Ricca V, Mannucci E, Moretti S, Di Bernardo M, Zucchi T, Cabras PL, et al. Screening for binge eating disorder in obese outpatients. Compr Psychiatry. 2000;41(2):111–5. https://doi.org/10.1016/s0010-440x(00)90143-3.
20. Allison KC, Crow SJ, Reeves RR, West DS, Foreyt JP, Dilillo VG, et al. Binge eating disorder and night eating syndrome in adults with type 2 diabetes. Obesity (Silver Spring, Md). 2007;15(5):1287–93. https://doi.org/10.1038/oby.2007.150.
21. Fairburn CG, Doll HA, Welch SL, Hay PJ, Davies BA, O'Connor ME. Risk factors for binge eating disorder: a community-based, case-control study. Arch Gen Psychiatry. 1998;55(5):425–32. https://doi.org/10.1001/archpsyc.55.5.425.
22. Mahmoud R, Kimonis V, Butler MG. Genetics of obesity in humans: a clinical review. Int J Mol Sci. 2022;23(19). https://doi.org/10.3390/ijms231911005.
23. Hrabosky JI, White MA, Masheb RM, Grilo CM. Physical activity and its correlates in treatment-seeking obese patients with binge eating disorder. Int J Eat Disord. 2007;40(1):72–6. https://doi.org/10.1002/eat.20323.
24. Brownell KD, Puhl RM, Schwartz MB, Rudd L. Weight bias: nature, consequences, and remedies. New York: Guilford Press; 2005.
25. Dovidio JF, Penner LA, Calabrese SK, Pearl RL. Physical health disparities and stigma: race, sexual orientation, and body weight. The Oxford handbook of stigma, discrimination, and health; 2018. p. 29–51.
26. Puhl RM, Andreyeva T, Brownell KD. Perceptions of weight discrimination: prevalence and comparison to race and gender discrimination in America. Int J Obes (Lond). 2008;32(6):992–1000. https://doi.org/10.1038/ijo.2008.22.
27. Durso LE, Latner JD. Understanding self-directed stigma: development of the weight bias internalization scale. Obesity. 2008;16(Suppl 2):S80–6. https://doi.org/10.1038/oby.2008.448.
28. Lillis J, Luoma JB, Levin ME, Hayes SC. Measuring weight self-stigma: the weight self-stigma questionnaire. Obesity. 2010;18(5):971–6. https://doi.org/10.1038/oby.2009.353.
29. Pearl RL, Bach C, Wadden TA. Development of a cognitive-behavioral intervention for internalized weight stigma. J Contemp Psychother. 2023;53(2):165–72. https://doi.org/10.1007/s10879-022-09543-w.
30. Himmelstein MS, Puhl RM, Quinn DM. Intersectionality: an understudied framework for addressing weight stigma. Am J Prev Med. 2017;53(4):421–31. https://doi.org/10.1016/j.amepre.2017.04.003.
31. Marshall RD, Latner JD, Masuda A. Internalized weight bias and disordered eating: the mediating role of body image avoidance and drive for thinness. Front Psychol. 2019;10:2999. https://doi.org/10.3389/fpsyg.2019.02999.
32. Pearl RL, Puhl RM, Lessard LM, Himmelstein MS, Foster GD. Prevalence and correlates of weight bias internalization in weight management: a multinational study. SSM Popul Health. 2021;13:100755. https://doi.org/10.1016/j.ssmph.2021.100755.

33. Pearl RL, Wadden TA, Hopkins CM, Shaw JA, Hayes MR, Bakizada ZM, et al. Association between weight bias internalization and metabolic syndrome among treatment-seeking individuals with obesity. Obesity. 2017;25(2):317–22. https://doi.org/10.1002/oby.21716.
34. Pearl RL, Dovidio JF. Experiencing weight bias in an unjust world: impact on exercise and internalization. Health Psychol. 2015;34(7):741–9. https://doi.org/10.1037/hea0000178.
35. Himmelstein MS, Puhl RM, Pearl RL, Pinto AM, Foster GD. Coping with weight stigma among adults in a commercial weight management sample. Int J Behav Med. 2020;27(5):576–90. https://doi.org/10.1007/s12529-020-09895-4.
36. Calugi S, Segattini B, Cattaneo G, Chimini M, Dalle Grave A, Dametti L, et al. Weight bias internalization and eating disorder psychopathology in treatment-seeking patients with obesity. Nutrients. 2023;15(13). https://doi.org/10.3390/nu15132932.
37. Carels RA, Wott CB, Young KM, Gumble A, Koball A, Oehlhof MW. Implicit, explicit, and internalized weight bias and psychosocial maladjustment among treatment-seeking adults. Eat Behav. 2010;11(3):180–5. https://doi.org/10.1016/j.eatbeh.2010.03.002
38. Bandura A. Social foundations of thought and action: a social cognitive theory. Englewood Cliffs: Prentice-Hall; 1986.

CBT for BED: An Overview

3

Abstract

Cognitive behaviour therapy (CBT) for binge-eating disorder (BED) integrates the strategies and procedures from both enanched CBT (CBT-E) for eating disorders and personalized CBT for obesity. Unlike treatments based on the "disease model", which address the patient's illness (e.g., BED), CBT for BED is based on the "psychological model"; it targets, in a personalized and flexible way, specific cognitive-behavioural processes that maintain binge-eating episodes and excessive and dysregulated eating and, in some patients, clinical obesity. The treatment, delivered in three steps, is collaborative, adaptable, and highly personalized. The therapist and patient work together as a team (collaborative empiricism), and the patient is encouraged to participate actively in the treatment process and to make treatment a priority. CBT for BED is an individual treatment, but, with the patient's prior consent, significant others can be involved in creating an optimal environment for change and helping the patient to implement some of the treatment procedures.

The term cognitive behaviour therapy (CBT) refers to a class of psychological treatments that are based on two interconnected premises: (i) cognitive mechanisms (beliefs and thoughts) and behaviours play a fundamental role in maintaining the problem; (ii) treatment must address these mechanisms, among other things. The strategies and procedures used as part of CBT depend on the issues to be addressed. CBT is mainly effective in treating clinical depression, anxiety disorders, and eating disorders.

CBT for binge-eating disorder (BED) is a specific form of CBT developed to help patients tackle their binge-eating episodes and associated psychopathology and, if indicated, achieve, accept, and sustain a healthy and reasonable weight loss. These objectives are pursued by addressing the factors that maintain BED (see

R. Dalle Grave et al., *Cognitive Behavior Therapy for Binge Eating Disorder*,
https://doi.org/10.1007/978-3-031-71456-6_3

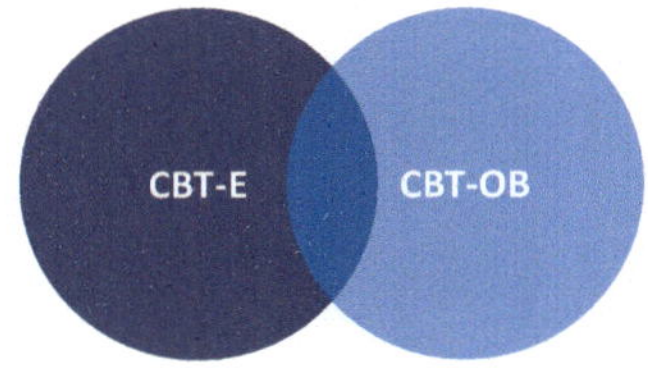

Fig. 3.1 Cognitive behavioural therapy (CBT) for binge-eating disorder (BED) integrates enhanced CBT (CBT-E) for eating disorders with personalized CBT for obesity (CBT-OB)

Chap. 2) through a personalized series of dedicated modules, incorporating two evidence-based interventions (Fig. 3.1).

1. Enhanced CBT (CBT-E) [1, 2] for eating disorders. This was developed for adults by the Centre for Research on Eating Disorders at Oxford (CREDO) [3] and for adolescents by our clinical team [1]. It is currently the most effective available option for treating binge-eating episodes and associated eating-disorder psychopathology [4], and is recommended for the treatment of both BED and bulimia nervosa by most international guidelines [5].
2. Personalized CBT for obesity (CBT-OB) [6]. Research shows that this treatment, also devised by our team [6], produces a healthy weight loss, ranging from 5% to 15%, in 70% of patients with clinical obesity (see Sect. 4.3.1 and Table 4.4 for the definition) [7–9]. Available data indicate that a 5% weight loss is associated with a reduction in cardiovascular risk factors and can prevent the onset of type 2 diabetes in individuals with prediabetes [10, 11]. A 10% weight loss reduces the risk of cardiovascular mortality [12], and 10–15% weight loss can lead to remission in type 2 diabetes in individuals who have had the condition for less than 6 years [13], as well as hepatic steatosis and obstructive sleep apnoea, and improves their quality of life [10].

3.1 Treatment Characteristics

CBT for BED is a treatment designed to address the cognitive behavioural processes that maintain BED a personalized way. It is effective irrespective of gender, and patients do not need special skills to explore and master their own psychological issues. Indeed, sometimes the most challenging patients to help are those who tend to theorize about their emotional experiences to control them, without making the necessary behavioural changes. For this reason, the treatment is practical in nature, with the patient being asked to complete homework and tasks between sessions. CBT for BED was designed as a comprehensive intervention, and should not be combined with other forms of psychotherapy. It is an adapted form of CBT, and like other empirically supported forms of CBT, it is a time-limited treatment that targets the processes that maintain a patient's specific problems. Unlike treatments based on the "disease model", which aim to treat a patient's illness (in this case BED), CBT for BED is based on the "psychological model", which, instead, uses a personalized and flexible series of modules to target specific cognitive-behavioural processes. These processes underlie and entrench binge-eating episodes and excessive, dysregulated eating and, in some patients, clinical obesity.

CBT for BED never adopts "prescriptive" procedures. In other words, the patients are never asked to do things they do not agree to do, because this only increases their resistance to change. Hence the therapist aims to build a collaborative relationship with the patient so that they can work together as a team to address the processes maintaining the patient's eating disorder. All procedures have been designed to actively involve a patient in all phases of their treatment, from the decision to start to identifying which problems to address and which strategies to adopt to this end. This is to give patients a feel of being in control, empowering them to actively participate in making changes and working collaboratively with their therapist to address their disorder, as per the tenets of collaborative empiricism.

Indeed, the key strategy in CBT for BED, as with other forms of CBT, is for the therapist and patient to work together to create a personalized formulation. This is essentially a diagram that illustrates the main processes maintaining a patient's binge-eating episodes and, if indicated, clinical obesity (according to cognitive behavioural theory), and therefore the mechanisms that the treatment is designed to target. As well as a mutual learning tool, it provides an individualized "road map" for treatment, and can be amended to deal with any processes emerging during the course of therapy. Thus, it is the basis for a tailor-made intervention addressing the maintenance mechanisms found to be operating in an individual patient via a sequential but flexible set of cognitive behavioural strategies and procedures integrated with patient education. Simpler procedures are preferred over more complex ones, with the treatment being guided by the "principle of parsimony" (it is better to do a few things well than many things badly).

As with other forms of CBT, continuous monitoring and completing strategically planned homework assignments are of paramount importance. Since these can create anxiety in some cases, the therapist, in addition to being empathetic, must be firm when necessary to ensure that these are effectively implemented. Although CBT for BED relies on a variety of generic behavioural and cognitive strategies (e.g., to address cognitive biases such as dichotomous thinking and selective attention), it differs from other forms of CBT in that it does not involve journalling dysfunctional thoughts. However, the last column of the patient's daily monitoring record (Fig. A1.1 in Appendix 1) can be used by them to record any events, thoughts, and emotions that influence their eating or they consider important, even if not related to eating. CBT for BED also differs from other forms of CBT in that it does not make much use of cognitive restructuring techniques or directly address automatic thoughts, assumptions, core beliefs, or schemas. Finally, although the treatment includes exploratory questions to help the patient clarify their thinking, it does not utilize Socratic dialogue, and no reference is made to "food addiction".

Instead, CBT for BED focuses on patients learning to decentre from their eating-disorder mindset and accept a reasonable weight. For this reason, it stimulates patients to become interested in understanding how their eating problem works and reinforces itself. To this end, the patient is encouraged to observe, using real-time self-monitoring, how the processes included in their personalized formulation

Table 3.1 General features of CBT for BED

A personalized and flexible treatment addressing key cognitive-behavioural processes that maintain binge-eating episodes and clinical obesity.
The therapist and patient work together as a team (collaborative empiricism).
The patient is empowered by encouraging them to participate actively in the treatment process and to make their treatment a priority.
Simpler procedures are preferred over more complex ones, as per the principle of parsimony.
To achieve cognitive change, the patient is encouraged to make specific behavioural modifications and analyze the effects and implications of these on their thinking.
The patient is encouraged to observe themself and identify cognitive and behavioural obstacles to a healthy long-term eating and weight-control lifestyle.
To forestall relapse, the patient is helped to identify the stimuli that reactivate their eating-disorder mindset and quickly decentre from the latter.

operate in their real life. To achieve cognitive change, the patient is prompted to make gradual modifications to their behaviour, and then to co-analyze the effects and implications of the same on their way of thinking. In the more advanced stages of treatment, when the main eating-disorder maintenance mechanisms have been disrupted, the therapy is designed to help the patient to recognize the first signs of reactivation of their eating-disorder mindset and to quickly decentre from it with a view to forestalling relapse.

Table 3.1 outlines the main features of CBT for BED.

3.2 The Goals

The main aim of CBT for BED is to help the patient stop binge eating and achieve, accept, and maintain a reasonable and healthy weight. This will involve the following therapeutic goals:

1. Engaging the patient actively in the treatment and decision to change
2. Eradicating the psychological and behavioural characteristics of the eating disorder
3. Correcting the mechanisms maintaining the eating disorder
4. Regularizing eating and addressing any emerging obstacles to achieving, accepting, and maintaining a reasonable, healthy weight
5. Making sure the changes are lasting.

3.3 The Steps

After the initial assessment and preparation sessions, the treatment is delivered across three main steps. The programme also includes mid-course review session (Fig. 3.2). With the exception of Step One, which has a fixed duration and standard content for all patients, the length of and modules covered by the rest of the

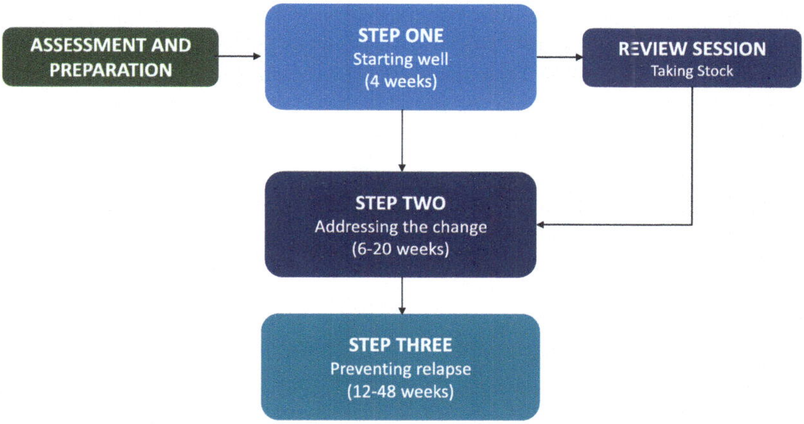

Fig. 3.2 The map of CBT for BED

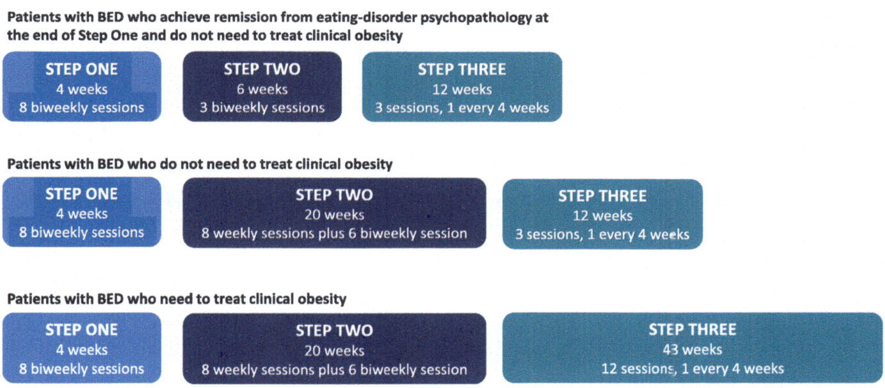

Fig. 3.3 The three possible durations of CBT for BED according to the patient's need or wish to lose weight and their response to treatment

treatment are flexible and personalized (Fig. 3.3). In summary, CBT for BED has three possible durations, according to the patient's need or wish to lose weight and their response to treatment (Fig. 3.3). The general structure of the programme is as follows:

Assessment and Preparation, which has the twin goals of assessing the nature and the severity of the eating disorder and associated clinical obesity (if they are present), and engaging the patients in the decision to change and start the treatment.

Step One: Starting Well aims to (i) increase the mutual understanding of the cognitive behavioural mechanisms that maintain a patient's BED, (ii) reduce their preoccupation with weight, (iii) reduce the frequency of their binge-eating episodes, and (iv) encourage them to adopt an active lifestyle. Note that it does not address weight loss, and any attempt to lose weight is discouraged at this stage. This step of the treatment lasts 4 weeks and involves two sessions per week.

Review Session: Taking Stock is scheduled for the end of Step One. It is devoted to (i) reviewing progress made in the first 4 weeks, (ii) identifying any obstacles to treatment, (iii) reviewing the personal formulation, and (iv) planning the next step.

Step Two: Addressing the Change is when patients start to tackle the maintenance mechanisms operating in their own individual manifestation of BED. The procedures begun in Step One are continued, and the treatment is personalized with the use of one or more of the following modules, as applicable:

- Healthy Weight Loss
- Events, Moods, and Eating
- Dysfunctional Dieting
- Overvaluation of Shape and Weight
- Unrealistic Weight Goals
- Internalized Weight Stigma
- Setbacks and Mindsets
- Maintenance Preparation

The duration of this Step will depend on the number of modules that are to be implemented and the rapidity of a patient's recovery. In most patients it takes about 20 weeks, and includes one session weekly for the first 2 months and then one session every 2 weeks. In patients who achieve early remission from their eating-disorder psychopathology and do not need to treat clinical obesity, however, Step Two includes only the Setbacks and Mindsets and Maintenance Preparation modules, and can be delivered in three biweekly sessions. The Healthy Weight Loss module can be associated with incretin-based weight-loss drugs (e.g., liraglutide, semaglutide, tirzepatide) in selected patients (see Chap. 12).

Step Three: Preventing Relapse has the aims of preventing binge eating from recurring and maintaining a healthy weight. It generally lasts 48 weeks and involves one session every 4 weeks. However, in patients who chose not to address weight loss during Step Two, Step Three is delivered over 3-monthly sessions and is focused on preventing binge-eating relapse.

3.4 Session Structure

Each session lasts 50 minutes and is structured as follows:

- Collaboratively weighing
- Reviewing the monitoring record and EPCL–BED (Eating Problem Checklist for BED, see Part 2 for details)
- Establishing the agenda (the topics to be addressed during the session)
- Implementing the agenda
- Agreeing on homework, summarizing the session and setting the next appointment

At helpful intervals and with the patient's prior agreement, joint sessions with the patient and their significant other(s) can be scheduled after individual sessions. These should last 15–20 minutes and aim to recruit them as "helpers", educating them on how to create a home environment conducive to change and facilitate the patient's implementation of certain treatment procedures.

3.5 The Role of the Patient

The patient is encouraged to play an active role both in and between sessions, and the treatment has little to no chance of success if they are not actively involved. Another attitude that CBT for BED advises the patient to adopt is to consider treatment a priority, akin to a new job or baby, for example. They should ascribe to the following motto: "*It's hard, but it will be worth it*". To reinforce the importance that the treatment should have in their life, the patient should be told that it is fundamental that each appointment start and end on time. They should be encouraged to arrive a little early (about 10–15 minutes before each session) to give them time to get comfortable, relax, and prepare things to discuss in the session. The patient is advised that they will need to work together with their therapist, as a team, to address their eating problem. Together, they will agree from time to time on specific tasks that the patient will have to undertake to carry out between one session and the next. Such tasks are essential and must be given absolute priority. It is precisely what the patient does between sessions that will allow the treatment to work. Finally, it is recommended that the patient avoid any interruptions to the programme so as not to interrupt the necessary therapeutic momentum.

3.6 The Role of Significant Others

CBT for BED is an individual treatment, and significant others of adult patients (friends, partners, or parents) are seen only if the patient agrees that their involvement will likely be helpful [2]. Generally, we plan three or four joint sessions of about 15 minutes in nearly one-third of our patients. When significant others are recruited, their role is simply as "helpers", supporting the patient to effect change. Typically, joint meetings with significant others are scheduled immediately after an individual session. Overall, support that patients may like to receive from significant others can be divided into two main categories [14]: (i) creating an optimal environment to facilitate patient change and (ii) helping to implement some of the treatment procedures.

The same principles apply to the treatment of adolescents, except for the fact that parents are always involved, given the age and circumstances of these patients. Parents are seen alone for a 50-minute session in the first week of treatment, and periodically in joint meetings with the adolescent and the therapist at the end of a patient's individual session [1]. The aims of the parents-only session are to assess the family environment, educate the parents about their adolescent child's eating disorder and the processes maintaining it (with reference to the personal formulation), address any self-blame, and stress the importance of creating an optimal family environment.

3.7 The Therapist's Prerequisites and Role

Therapists who wish to practice CBT for BED must ascribe to the cognitive behavioural perspective of the processes that maintain binge-eating episodes and hinder weight loss and maintenance, and have a detailed understanding of the treatment and personalized formulation (i.e., the case conceptualization). They should also be familiar with the psychopathology underlying BED, the physiopathology of obesity, and the associated psychosocial and medical complications. Preferably, the therapist should have experience working with patients with eating disorders and clinical obesity, and be able to recognize and address the medical complications of clinical obesity or have access to other specialists who can.

Clinical experience is the most important factor. Therapists should be proactive and empathetic but also firm when needed. They should devote their efforts to working collaboratively with the patient, keeping them involved in treatment and lifestyle changes, and taking care to avoid any interruptions in treatment. CBT for BED training advises therapists not to adopt overt or subtle weight stigma-reinforcing attitudes or behaviours. Some patients report being dissatisfied with their poor communication with health professionals when receiving advice on weight loss and change, when perceiving stigmatizing and discriminatory attitudes towards them. Hence, the therapist should be scrupulously aware of the language they use with their patients. Terms such as "morbid obesity" and "fat", must be avoided, as they cause patients, especially people with clinical obesity, to feel stigmatized. However, it is important to underline that there is not one universally preferred term for people living in larger bodies. Health professionals should discuss preferred language with each patient, adopting terms that the individual themself chooses or finds acceptable when discussing clinical obesity. This can positively influence patient care. Indeed, various studies have shown that a patient's perception that the therapist has weight-related biases decreases their motivation to lose weight, increases short-term calorie consumption, and worsens treatment outcome.

These indications are added to those provided by the Rudd Center for Food Policy & Obesity (http://www.uconnruddcenter.org), which recommends "always putting the person before the disease (People-First Language)" when describing a person with obesity. For example, instead of saying, "*There are a lot of obese people*", say, "*There are a lot of people with obesity*". Labelling a person as their illness dehumanizes the individual, and it is not appropriate to say that a person is obese when they have obesity, just as it is customary not to say that a person is cancerous when they have cancer.

3.8 Therapeutic Setting

An appropriate office environment is essential for managing patients with BED and obesity effectively. Patients should be made to feel comfortable, and any situations that might create embarrassment preventatively addressed. Attention to the practical needs of patients demonstrates understanding and sensitivity. Some suggestions for establishing an appropriate therapeutic environment for these patients are as follows:

- The office should be barrier-free (e.g., no steep hills or long flights of stairs), easily accessible by public transport, and close to a parking space.
- Chairs in the waiting and treatment rooms should be sturdy, spacious, and without armrests.
- Scales should be suitable for patients with obesity, with a large and robust base.
- Blood pressure monitors should have a wide bracelet.
- All office staff (doctors, psychologists, dieticians, interns, secretaries, etc.) should be empathetic, respectful, and non-judgmental toward patients with clinical obesity (see above).
- Information materials and manuals on BED and obesity should be carefully worded and easily accessible for patients.

References

1. Dalle Grave R, Calugi S. Cognitive behavior therapy for adolescents with eating disorders. New York: Guilford Press; 2020.
2. Fairburn CG. Cognitive behavior therapy and eating disorders. New York: Guilford Press; 2008.
3. Fairburn CG, Cooper Z, Shafran R. Cognitive behaviour therapy for eating disorders: a "transdiagnostic" theory and treatment. Behav Res Ther. 2003;41(5):509–28. https://doi.org/10.1016/s0005-7967(02)00088-8.
4. Linardon J, Wade TD, de la Piedad GX, Brennan L. The efficacy of cognitive-behavioral therapy for eating disorders: a systematic review and meta-analysis. J Consult Clin Psychol. 2017;85(11):1080–94. https://doi.org/10.1037/ccp0000245.
5. National Guideline Alliance. Eating disorders: recognition and treatment. London: National Institute for Health and Care Excellence (UK); 2017 May. (NICE Guideline, No. 69.). London: 2017.
6. Dalle Grave R, Sartirana M, El Ghoch M, Calugi S. Treating obesity with personalized cognitive behavioral therapy. Cham: Springer; 2018.
7. Dalle Grave R, Calugi S, Gavasso I, El Ghoch M, Marchesini G. A randomized trial of energy-restricted high-protein versus high-carbohydrate, low-fat diet in morbid obesity. Obesity (Silver Spring). 2013;21(9):1774–81. https://doi.org/10.1002/oby.20320.
8. Dalle Grave R, Calugi S, Bosco G, Valerio L, Valenti C, El Ghoch M, et al. Personalized group cognitive behavioural therapy for obesity: a longitudinal study in a real-world clinical setting. Eat Weight Disord. 2018;25(2). https://doi.org/10.1007/s40519-018-0593-z.
9. Calugi S, Ruocco A, El Ghoch M, Andrea C, Geccherle E, Sartori F, et al. Residential cognitive-behavioral weight-loss intervention for obesity with and without binge-eating disorder: a prospective case-control study with five-year follow-up. Int J Eat Disord. 2016;49(7):723–30. https://doi.org/10.1002/eat.22549.

10. Ryan DH, Yockey SR. Weight loss and improvement in comorbidity: differences at 5%, 10%, 15%, and over. Curr Obes Rep. 2017;6(2):187–94. https://doi.org/10.1007/s13679-017-0262-y.
11. Knowler WC, Barrett-Connor E, Fowler SE, Hamman RF, Lachin JM, Walker EA, et al. Reduction in the incidence of type 2 diabetes with lifestyle intervention or metformin. N Engl J Med. 2002;346(6):393–403. https://doi.org/10.1056/NEJMoa012512.
12. Gregg EW, Jakicic JM, Blackburn G, Bloomquist P, Bray GA, Clark JM, et al. Association of the magnitude of weight loss and changes in physical fitness with long-term cardiovascular disease outcomes in overweight or obese people with type 2 diabetes: a post-hoc analysis of the Look AHEAD randomised clinical trial. Lancet Diabetes Endocrinol. 2016;4(11):913–21. https://doi.org/10.1016/s2213-8587(16)30162-0.
13. Lean ME, Leslie WS, Barnes AC, Brosnahan N, Thom G, McCombie L, et al. Primary care-led weight management for remission of type 2 diabetes (DiRECT): an open-label, cluster-randomised trial. Lancet. 2018;391(10120):541–51. https://doi.org/10.1016/s0140-6736(17)33102-1.
14. Dalle Grave R, el Khazen C. Cognitive behaviour therapy for eating disorders in young people: a parents' guide. London: Routledge; 2022.

4 Assessment, Preparation, and Medical Management

Abstract

The assessment and preparation of the patient about to start cognitive behavior therapy (CBT) for binge-eating disorder (BED) has three main goals. The first is to assess the nature and severity of the eating-disorder psychopathology using a data-driven approach. Information should be gathered on current status (i.e., current body weight, height, waist circumference, eating behaviour; levels of physical activity, body image, and quality of life), weight and eating disorder history, any previous treatments for obesity and eating disorder (including unmanaged efforts to lose weight), weight goals and reasons for wanting to lose weight, barriers to weight loss, and personal and family medical histories. The second goal is to engage the patients in the treatment. To this end, the therapist should adopt an engaging style, educating patients on BED, clinical obesity, and CBT for BED, assessing their readiness to change, actively involving them in the decision to effect change, and to make the programme a priority. One session is usually devoted to assessment and preparation, at the end of which a decision has to be made on how best to proceed. With ambivalent patients, one additional assessment interview may be scheduled to make a further attempt to engage them in the decision to start the treatment. Non-medical therapists preparing patients for CBT for BED should always refer them to a physician for the assessment and management of physical complications associated with BED and clinical obesity.

The assessment and preparation of the patient for cognitive behavior therapy (CBT) for binge-eating disorder (BED) generally takes place in one session, which has three main objectives: (i) to assess the nature and severity of a patient's eating-disorder psychopathology, (ii) to engage the patient in treatment, and (iii) to decide how best to proceed. First impressions are crucial. A positive encounter can involve even the most ambivalent patient, while a negative meeting can have the opposite effect and may lead to the decision not to start treatment.

R. Dalle Grave et al., *Cognitive Behavior Therapy for Binge Eating Disorder*, https://doi.org/10.1007/978-3-031-71456-6_4

4.1 Developing a Trusting and Collaborative Therapeutic Relationship

A key strategy of CBT for BED is to establish a relationship with their patient that should be characterized by both cooperation and mutual trust. It is vital that the ground for this relationship is laid in the assessment and preparation session, and that it continues throughout treatment. With this in mind, the therapist should warmly welcome the patient and put them at ease. It should always be kept in mind that people with clinical obesity (see Sect. 4.3.1 for the definition) may be somewhat defensive or fearful, as they are often stigmatized and judged critically, not only by other individuals but also by health professionals [1].

A good "icebreaker" question is to ask the patient who advised them to attend the meeting. This question helps create an empathetic bond, and can foster the patient's willingness to share information about their problems. Immediately afterward, the patient should be asked why they actually came to the assessment session: a question that helps shed light on whether their main goal is to lose weight or to address their eating disorder. This information allows the therapist to adapt the diagnostic process accordingly.

The patient should be given as much time as they need to describe their problems, without overloading them with questions and questionnaires, and to answer any questions they may have.

4.2 Assessing the Nature and Severity of BED

After putting the patient at ease, the therapist should take a medical and psychological history, focusing in particular on assessing their eating-disorder psychopathology and body weight history. Table 4.1 provides a list of points that are helpful to cover. The interview should begin by gathering general personal information and detecting any social circumstances that might affect the treatment. Since binge-eating episodes are often kept secret, some patients may be hesitant, embarrassed, or reluctant to talk about them, and are seeking treatment for their weight or other psychological issues (e.g., depression, anxiety) rather than the eating disorder [2]. Others may not know that binge eating is an understandable behaviour that is part of a specific, treatable, eating disorder; they just know they feel bad about it. Patients' lack of awareness of having a distinct eating disorder stems in part from the fact that even clinicians poorly understand BED. In a U.S. survey of 23,396 adults, for example, only 3.2 percent of those who had met the diagnostic criteria for BED in the previous 12 months (1.5 percent of the sample) had received this diagnosis from their physician [3]. Another survey of 278 U.S. physicians (psychiatrists, family physicians, internists, gynaecologists) found that 10 percent did not screen their patients' eating habits, even if they had symptoms of an eating disorder. In addition, more than half did not use the BED diagnostic criteria and a quarter did not know that it was a distinct eating disorder [4].

Table 4.1 List of points to be investigated

Personal information
Age
Race
Marital status and attitude of the spouse or significant other toward the treatment
Education
Living situation (household members)
Children
Employment and working hours
Interests
Body weight history
Weight at different stages of life (birth, menarche or puberty, at age 20, before and after pregnancy, menopause)
Minimum and maximum weight
Age at onset of obesity
Change in weight over the past year
Events associated with weight gain
Eating disorder history
Age of onset of binge-eating episodes (lasting at least 3 months)
Weight at the time of onset of binge-eating episodes
Precipitating factors (12 months before onset)
Dieting to lose weight and change body shape
Life events
Mood changes
Other
Previous eating disorders (e.g., anorexia nervosa, bulimia nervosa, other eating disorders): type and age of onset
Any change in eating habits (e.g., periods of extreme dietary restriction) or unhealthy weight-control behaviours (e.g., self-induced vomiting, misuse of laxatives and diuretics, use of weight-loss medications) after onset
Previous treatments for obesity
Nature and duration
Overall adherence
Maximum weight loss and degree of satisfaction
Duration of weight loss maintenance
Possible reasons for weight regain
Number of weight-loss and regain cycles
Previous treatments for eating disorders
Nature and duration
Overall adherence
Outcome
Current status
Current weight and height (measured) and calculation of body mass index (BMI)
Waist circumference

(continued)

Table 4.1 (continued)

Menstrual status (in women)
Eating habits (e.g., portion size, food choice, and frequency of meals)
Binge-eating episodes: frequency and triggers
Physical activity (nature and frequency of lifestyle activities and formal exercise)
Extreme weight-control behaviours (e.g., self-induced vomiting, laxatives and/or diuretics misuse): frequency and triggers
Alcohol and/or substance misuse: frequency and triggers
Body checking and avoidance: frequency and triggers
Importance of shape and weight in self-evaluation
Effects and binge-eating episodes and body weight on physical health, psychological well-being, social functioning, and school and/or work performance
Weight goals/expectations
Dream weight, desired weight and maximum acceptable weight
Reasons for wanting to lose weight
Obstacles to change
Personal (e.g., low motivation, low self-efficacy, deflected mood, use of food to manage emotions)
External (e.g., family difficulties, stress at work, exposure to food at work)
Personal and family medical history
Current and past medical and psychiatric comorbidity
Current medications
Family medical and psychiatric history

The next step is to reconstruct a detailed history of the patients' eating-disorder psychopathology and body weight. The aim is to understand if there is, as often occurs, a relationship between the two. As mentioned, it is vital to ask patients about their eating habits in a way that does not make them feel stigmatized, allowing them to describe their behaviour calmly and without fear of being judged. Questions should focus on discovering whether the binge-eating episodes appeared after a period of dieting and/or in association with life events and associated mood changes, whether they led to weight gain, and whether they were preceded by other forms of eating disorder (e.g., anorexia nervosa, bulimia nervosa, other eating disorders).

The next step is to ask the patient about the nature of any previous attempts at treatment for obesity and/or eating disorder(s). Because it is common for the patient to repeat the same behavioural patterns, this information can help both the therapist and the patient focus on specific, potentially recurring problems.

The patient's current state must be carefully assessed. This involves asking for permission to measure their weight and height, and calculate BMI. The waist circumference must also be measured (at the level of the iliac crest of the pelvis) because, if it is high (>102 cm in men and >88 cm in women) it is associated with an increased risk of type 2 diabetes, dyslipidaemias, hypertension, and cardiovascular disease [5, 6].

A short-term history of eating behaviour should also be noted, asking the patient to remember their eating-behaviour patterns over the previous 24 days (i.e., what they ate, how often, and how they rate their portion sizes). The therapist should also take the opportunity to enquire about any binge-eating episodes, extreme weight-control behaviours (e.g., self-induced vomiting or misuse of laxatives or diuretics) and/or alcohol and substance misuse. A physical activity history should also be collected, and the patient should be asked if they have ever adopted an active lifestyle or practiced formal exercise.

Then, the patient's attitude toward their physical appearance should be explored, assessing the frequency and nature of several key behavioural expressions of negative body image, such as body checking and avoidance, and the importance of shape and weight in their self-evaluation. The patient should also be asked how their binge-eating episodes and obesity (if present) are affecting their health, psychological well-being, social functioning, and school and/or work performance [7].

Without making any comment, the therapist should also ask about the patient's personal weight goals and, if they would like to lose weight, the reasons. While these factors don't need to be addressed at this stage, our research indicates that unrealistic weight-loss expectations encourage the adoption of dysfunctional dieting, which can contribute to the maintenance of binge-eating episodes [8].

Analyzing the patient's perceived general barriers to change is also helpful. These can be internal (e.g., low motivation, low self-efficacy, low mood, and/or use of food to modulate mood) or external (e.g., difficulties within the family, stress at work, and/or exposure to food at work) [7].

The final step in this information-gathering stage is to accurately assess the patient's physical, psychological, and psychiatric medical history. In particular, the therapist should ask about past or present anxiety and mood disorders, as these are common among patients with BED, and can be a barrier to treatment if not adequately addressed. It is also essential to determine whether or not patients are taking medications that may contribute to weight gain, and whether a change in their weight trajectory is associated with taking a new medication [9]. If this association is observed, a drug not associated with weight gain or one producing weight loss should be considered (if possible) as an alternative treatment for the medical condition, involving the physician following the patient's medical condition (see Table 4.2) in this decision [10]. It is also essential to assess the patient's family history of medical and psychiatric conditions, especially the presence of a positive family history of obesity or eating disorders [9].

The initial assessment can be completed by asking the patient to fill in some self-report questionnaires. These can be used as a starting point to assess the effects of CBT for BED over time. In our clinical practice, for example, we use the following instruments at baseline, the end of treatment, and follow-up:

- Eating Disorder Examination Questionnaire (EDE-Q) [11, 12]. The EDE-Q is a 36-item self-report questionnaire used to assess a patient's eating-disorder psychopathology over the previous 28 days. It provides a global score based on four subscales designed to reflect the severity of the main features of eating-disorder psychopathology (Restraint, Eating Concern, Shape Concern, and Weight Concern). It also assesses key behavioural features of eating disorders, including

Table 4.2 Medications associated with weight gain and possible alternatives

Drug Class	Medications associated with weight gain	Alternative options to consider (weight neutral or associated with weight loss)
Antidiabetics	Insulin, glitazones/thiazolidinediones, sulfonylureas	Acarbose, DPP-4 inhibitors, GLP-1 analogues, pramlintide, SGLT2 inhibitors
Antihypertensive	Atenolol, doxazosin, metoprolol, propranolol, terazosin	ACE inhibitors, ARB, carvedilol, daxozin, nebivolol
Steroid hormones	Glucocorticoids, progestogens	Lowest dosage of glucocorticoids to control obesity-associated disease, NSAIDs
Antipsychotics	Clozapine, olanzapine, quetiapine, risperidone	Aripiprazole, ziprasidone, paliperidone, lurasidone, asenapine
Antidepressants	MAOIs (e.g., phenelzine), mirtazapine, SSRIs (citalopram, fluoxetine >1 year, paroxetine, sertraline >1 year), TCAs (amitriptyline, imipramine, nortriptyline)	Fluoxetine <1 year, sertraline <1 year, bupropion)
Neurological agents	Carbamazepine, gabapentin, lithium pregabalin, valproate,	Lamotrigine, levetiracetam, phenytoin, topiramate, zonisamide
Antihistamines	Diphenhydramine, other antihistamines	Short-term use
Contraceptives	High-dose oestrogen–progestogen combinations, medroxyprogesterone acetate	IUDs, low-dose oestrogen–progestogen combinations

ACE angiotensin-converting enzyme, *ARBs* angiotensin receptor blockers, *DPP-4* dipeptidyl peptidase 4, *GLP-1* glucagon-like peptide-1, *MAOIs* monoamine oxidase inhibitors, *NSAIDs* nonsteroidal anti-inflammatory drugs, *SGLT2* sodium-glucose transport protein 2, *SSRIs* selective serotonin-reuptake inhibitors, *TCAs* tricyclic antidepressants

binge eating, self-induced vomiting, laxative misuse, diuretic misuse, and excessive exercising.

- Clinical Impairment Assessment (CIA) [13, 14]. The CIA is a self-report instrument that assesses the severity of clinical impairment secondary to the eating-disorder psychopathology over the past 28 days. Its 16 items explore harm in areas of life that are typically affected by the psychopathology of eating disorders, namely mood and self-perception, cognitive functioning, interpersonal functioning, and occupational performance.

- Brief Symptom Inventory (BSI) [15]. The BSI is a 53-item self-report instrument that assesses psychological distress over the last 7 days. The Global Severity Index (GSI) is calculated based on the scores assigned to participants' responses.
- Short Form-36 (SF-36). The SF-36 is a 26-item generic health-related quality-of-life questionnaire [16, 17], incorporating questions about functioning in and satisfaction with various life domains. It assesses four domains related to the physical component of quality of life (Physical Functioning, Physical Role Functioning, Bodily Pain and General Health Perception) and four domains related to the seven mental components (Vitality, Social Role Functioning, Emotional Role Functioning and Mental Health).
- Weight Bias Internalization Scale (WBIS) [18, 19]. The WBIs uses a total of 11 items (e.g., "*I am less attractive than most other people because of my weight*", "*I hate myself because of my weight*"), rated on a seven-point Likert scale, to evaluate internalized weight bias, a construct associated with psychopathology and, as described in Chap. 2, maintenance of binge-eating episodes in a subgroup of patients. It is useful for screening patients for internalized weight stigma, a key component of their personal formulation (see Chap. 6) to be addressed during treatment (see Chap. 17).

We also use the Eating Disorder Examination interview (EDE 17.0D) [20, 21] to confirm the diagnosis of eating disorder according to the DSM-5. The EDE interview is designed to evaluate eating disorder psychopathology and behaviours over the 28 days before the interview is conducted. Scores of 0–6 are assigned to the behavioural symptoms (binge eating, self-induced vomiting, laxative misuse, diuretics misuse, excessive exercising, and food restriction) exhibited by individuals with eating disorders, and there is a specific module with diagnostic items for BED. EDE scores can be expressed on a global scale, but also through four specific subscales (Restraint, Eating Concern, Weight Concern, and Shape Concern), reflecting the respective cognitive features of eating disorders. We recommend that the EDE 17.0D be completed for all patients with BED, as it contains questions, designed to assess the presence of overvaluation of shape and weight (see Table 4.3), which, as described in Chap. 2, acts as an indicator of BED severity and a powerful maintenance mechanism of binge-eating episodes.

N.B. The English version of EDE 17.0D, EDE-Q, and CIA can be downloaded at this website https://www.cbte.co/for-professionals/measures/

Table 4.3 Eating Disorder Examination interview (EDE 17.0D) questions to assess the importance of weight and shape

1. Over the past four weeks, has your weight (the number on the scale) been important in influencing how you feel about (judge, think, evaluate) yourself as a person?
2. What about your shape? How has it compared in importance with your weight in influencing how you feel about yourself?
Since these concepts are quite complex, the following exploratory question should be asked to ensure that the patient understands the two diagnostic questions:
If you imagine the things that influence how you feel about (judge, think, evaluate) yourself—such as (your performance at work, being a parent, your marriage, how you get on with other people)—and put these things in order of importance, where does your weight fit in?
If the patient is denying that their weight and/or body shape is important but their behaviour suggests otherwise, the following two questions should be asked:
a) If, over the past four weeks, your weight had changed in any way, would this have affected how you felt about yourself?
b) Over the past four weeks, has it been important to you that your weight does not change? Have you been making sure that it does not change?
Then a score is assigned on a scale that includes seven points for each of the first two questions (1 and 2) as follows:
0 - No importance
1 -
2 - Some importance (definitely an aspect of self-evaluation)
3 -
4 - Moderate importance (definitely one of the main aspects of self-evaluation)
5 -
6 - Supreme importance (nothing is more important in the participant's scheme for self-evaluation)
If the patient scores ≥4 on one or both questions, they are considered to have overvaluation of shape and/or weight [22].

4.3 Medical Assessment

As mentioned, any medical conditions the patient may have must be treated by a medical doctor, preferably one who is familiar with CBT for BED and/or clinical obesity. However, the following paragraphs provide some general information for non-medical therapists on the medical assessment of patients with BED associated with clinical obesity.

4.3.1 Things Non-medical Therapists Should Keep in Mind

- The health and safety of patients with BED associated with clinical obesity is paramount and should never be overlooked or underestimated.
- Clinical obesity can be associated with several medical complications, and therapists should be aware of this.
- Non-medical therapists conducting the assessment and preparation phase should always refer patients to a physician so that their physical complications associated with clinical obesity can be safely assessed and treated.

- Non-medical therapists delivering CBT for BED associated with clinical obesity should ensure that patients have a physician who takes responsibility for their medical management. Therapists should exchange contact details with this doctor so they can get in touch if necessary.
- Most of the risk factors and complications associated with clinical obesity improve with a 5–10% weight reduction, normalization of eating habits, and adoption of an active lifestyle. However, in some cases, the doctor may prescribe medication for specific risk factors (e.g., high blood pressure, prediabetes or diabetes, hypercholesterolemia, hypertriglyceridemia) to manage the cardiovascular risk and enhance the effects of lifestyle modification.
- No specific laboratory or clinical tests are necessary to diagnose BED. However, for a diagnosis of clinical obesity, it is necessary to measure a patient's weight and height (to calculate BMI) and waist circumference. Medical assessment and several blood and instrumental tests are also warranted to distinguish clinical obesity from non-clinical obesity or higher BMI (see Table 4.4 for the definitions).

Table 4.4 Clinical obesity and non-clinical obesity

Obesity became recognized as a disease by several medical societies and countries between 2013 and 2022. The World Obesity Federation defines obesity as a "chronic relapsing progressive disease" [23] while the 2020 Canadian Clinical Practice Guidelines state that it is a "complex chronic disease in which abnormal or excess body fat (adiposity) impairs health increases the risk of long-term medical complications and reduces lifespan" [24].
However the BMI thresholds historically used to define obesity have been designed and studied as predictors of disease or future mortality in the population but not as measures of existing disease in a single individual [24]. For this reason the BMI threshold ≥30 cannot be used as the sole diagnostic indicator of obesity. Indeed individuals with BMI values in the "normal" range can present cardiometabolic metabolic complications commonly found in people with obesity (e.g. cardiovascular diseases type 2 diabetes) while some individuals with a BMI ≥30 do not have evidence of organ disease or functional limitations metabolic disorder or cardiovascular disease—including type 2 diabetes dyslipidaemia hypertension and atherosclerosis—or symptoms of physical disability nor psychosocial impairment. This condition is known as "metabolically healthy obesity" [25, 26]. There are also people with high BMI low adiposity and high muscle density (i.e. body builders/athletes in larger bodies). This means that BMI should not be used to diagnose clinical obesity and indicate treatment but merely to screen for obesity in the general population.
Hence the key aspect to consider in a patient is not weight per se but whether excess or abnormal body fat (adiposity) impairs health and psychological well-being. This frame of reference allows us to distinguish between three conditions [27]:
1. *Clinical obesity,* which is a chronic, systemic illness characterized by alterations in the function of tissues, organs (e.g., heart, lung, kidney, liver) or the individual (e.g., poor physical fitness, limitation of daily activities, physical disability, poor psychological well-being). Clinical obesity is commonly associated with several obesity-related medical and psychological comorbidities. This condition can be present also in individuals with a BMI ≤ 30.
2. *Non-clinical obesity*, sometimes referred to as "*pre-clinical obesity*", which is characterized by a state of excess adiposity, but the function of other tissues and organs is preserved (e.g., physically active female with a prevalent subcutaneous fat distribution, with a BMI of 33 kg/m^2, no physical symptoms, no cardiovascular risk factors, no self-esteem issues, and no functional limitations) Although not classed as a disease, this condition is a risk factor for developing clinical obesity, as well as several other non-communicable diseases [28].
3. *High BMI without obesity*, which is a condition characterized by a BMI ≥30 but high lean mass (as occurs in some athletes) and no excess fat mass.

4.3.2 Recommended Medical Tests

The laboratory and instrumental tests that should be administered to patients with BED and obesity before they start CBT for BED are as follows (N.B. non-medical therapists should not attempt to interpret the results of these tests; instead, they should delegate this task to the medical doctor treating the patient) [29]:

- Complete blood count with formula (to count white blood cells, red blood cells and platelets, the concentration of haemoglobin, and the haematocrit, i.e., the volume percentage of red blood cells)
- Alanine aminotransferase (ALT), aspartate aminotransferase (AST), gamma-glutamyl transferase (GGT) (to assess liver function)
- Creatinine, and glomerular filtration rate (GFR) (to assess kidney function)
- Potassium, sodium, calcium, magnesium, and phosphorus levels (to assess electrolyte status)
- Glucose, insulin, LDL and HDL cholesterol, and triglycerides (to assess cardiovascular risk)
- C-reactive protein and fibrinogen (to detect any inflammatory conditions)
- Thyroid-stimulating hormone (TSH) (to assess thyroid function)
- Vitamin D [25(OH)D] (to assess vitamin D levels)
- Urinalysis (to assess hydration status and detect urinary infections or other complications)
- Electrocardiogram (to assess any changes in heart rhythm)
- Systolic and diastolic blood pressure (to detect high blood pressure)
- Abdominal ultrasound (in case of suspected steatotic liver disease)
- Pelvic ultrasound (in case of suspected polycystic ovary syndrome)
- Epworth Sleepiness Scale and polysomnography (in case of suspected obstructive sleep apnoea syndrome)
- Bioelectrical impedance analysis or dual-energy X-ray absorptiometry (DEXA) (to measure body composition)

A physician should also assess whether the patients have an alteration of tissues or organs (e.g., heart, lung, kidney, liver) determined by obesity and/or obesity-related medical comorbidities.

N.B. The psychosocial and medical examination and tests permit detection of the presence of "clinical obesity" (see Table 4.5) or non-clinical (pre-clinical obesity)

Table 4.5 Features of clinical obesity

The presence of clinical obesity should be diagnosed when the patients have obesity-related comorbidities or alterations in the function of tissues, organs, or the individual
Alterations in the function of tissues, organs, or the individual
Deposition of ectopic fat (e.g., visceral, hepatic, epicardial, myocardial, pancreatic, muscular, or renal sinus levels) and/or or higher weight associated with one or more of the following features:
Low-grade inflammation
Hyperinsulinemia
Alteration of liver enzymes
Dyspnoea
Borderline hypertension
Impaired fasting glucose
Elevated liver enzymes
Aches/pains
Fatigue
Reduced mobility
Impaired quality of life
Inability to work or complete daily activities
Obesity-related medical comorbidities
Hypertension
Type 2 Diabetes
Sleep apnoea
PCOS
Osteoarthritis
Reflux disease
Obesity-related psychological comorbidities
Mood disorders
Anxiety disorders
Eating disorder

4.4 Engaging the Patient in the Decision to Change

CBT for BED does not include a long motivational pathway for involving a patient in the treatment because the treatment itself is intrinsically motivating. Indeed, by helping the patient to reduce the frequency of their binge-eating episodes over the first 4 weeks, it enhances their active engagement in both the programme and change. In addition, a patient generally engages when they feel they are being listened to and understood. Therefore, CBT for BED places great emphasis on adopting an engaging style (see Table 4.6, which is vital to establishing a trusting therapeutic relationship and the key to motivating change [7]. The approach to engaging the patient will vary based on their motivation levels, but in all cases, it must include conveying empathy, understanding and competence, and instilling hope.

Table 4.6 Tips for adopting an engaging style

Conceptualization of motivation. Motivation is a dynamic entity that waxes and wanes as personal, cognitive, behavioural, and environmental determinants change. For this reason, therapists should pay constant attention to the patient's motivation levels both during the engagement process and throughout treatment [7].
Collaborative therapeutic style. The therapist should adopt a collaborative style of delivering therapy rather than a directive approach [30]. The collaborative style of CBT is considered one of the main reasons for its greater success in engaging ambivalent patients, as compared to other interventions [31].
Showing empathy. Patients in general, and especially those with BED, who tend to receive frequent criticism of their weight and behaviour, appreciate a helpful therapist who shows interest in them as people.
Acceptance and change. The therapist should validate patient experiences within a balanced context of acceptance, change, firmness, and empathy [32].
Functional analysis. The therapist should engage each patient in a functional analysis of the potential advantages and disadvantages of treatment. Change is facilitated by communication that elicits the motivations and benefits of change [33].
Overcoming resistance. The therapist should not meet resistance with confrontation, but instead with a collaborative assessment of the variables involved in maintaining their unhealthy behaviour [33].
Supporting self-efficacy. Self-efficacy refers to a person's belief that they can adhere to a specific behaviour [34], and is important for achieving healthy behavioural change [35]. In the initial assessment interview, clinicians should already begin to promote self-efficacy by raising or fostering the hope that lifestyle changes and overcoming binge eating are achievable. During the programme, self-efficacy should be promoted by setting achievable tasks and collaboratively identifying the mechanisms maintaining the patient's eating disorder, establishing specific strategies and procedures to address them.
Being sensitive to weight stigma. Stigma does have an influence on a patient with clinical obesity's decision to start treatment [36]. Hence, the patient should never feel judged for their weight, and should receive all the respect and support they need [7]. As described in Chap. 3, it is strongly recommended that people-first language be used when describing or talking to a person with clinical obesity. Clinicians should reassure such patients that clinical obesity is not merely the product of a lack of willpower. Instead, it results from a complex interplay of genetic, epigenetic, environmental, emotional, cognitive, and behavioural factors that are only partially understood [37].
Inviting questions. The therapist should ask the patient if they have any concerns or questions. This approach will encourage engagement and foster the development of an open and empathetic therapeutic relationship [7].

Other strategies useful for engaging the patient in the decision to change are to ask them about their reasons and personal motivations for getting treatment, information about previous treatment attempts, and whether they feel ready to change. The patient should also be accurately informed about the goals, duration, organization, procedures, and potential outcomes of treatment [7].

4.5 Educating the Patient about BED and Clinical vs. Non-clinical Obesity

At this point in the interview, the therapist should ask the patient if they would like some information about their problem. If the answer is yes, as is usually the case, a helpful way to educate the patient is to design a "generic formulation", as in Chap. 2 Fig. 2.1, underlining, however, that their own "personal formulation" will be compiled during treatment. The generic formulation, which includes the main features and mechanisms of binge-eating episodes and clinical obesity, is used to explain that binge-eating episodes, overeating and dysregulated eating are usually triggered and maintained by events and associated mood changes and/or by the intermittent adoption of extreme and rigid dieting (i.e., dysfunctional dieting). In turn, these are often the result of preoccupation with shape and weight, which is intensified by the binge-eating episodes themselves.

Patients with clinical obesity should also be educated on their interaction with binge eating, explaining that binge eating promotes weight gain, which in turn contributes to the maintenance of binge eating through the following mechanisms: (i) creating negative mood states, often associated with internalized weight stigma, and (ii) intensifying preoccupation with shape and weight and often leading to the development of unrealistic weight goals, with the consequent intermittent adoption of dysfunctional dieting. Finally, reduced physical activity, a common consequence of weight gain, further contributes to increasing body weight.

We also educate patients that obesity is determined by an interplay between genetic predisposition, with an estimated heritability rate for BMI of between 40 and 70%; environmental factors and some learned habits. However, we underscore that a BMI $\geq$ 30, used as a threshold for obesity, has been designed and studied as a predictor of disease or future mortality in the population but not as a measure of existing disease in a single individual. Indeed, the key aspect to consider is not weight per se, but whether there are alterations in the function of tissues, organs or the individual due raised or excess body fat (adiposity). In presence of "clinical obesity" (see Table 4.4) [28], there is strong evidence that a reasonable weight loss (e.g., $\geq$5%) will produce improvements in most of its complications [38]. On the other hand, when higher body weight is not associated with health impairment (i.e., non-clinical obesity), weight loss could prevent the development of clinical obesity, but not necessarily reduce the risk of weight-related illnesses.

Finally, the patient should also be informed that while clinical obesity is a chronic disease, like diabetes, that requires the adoption of a persistent lifestyle change, complete remission of BED can be achieved through treatment.

4.6 Explaining the Nature of the Treatment

The next step, if CBT for BED is indicated, is to describe the treatment to the patient (see Chap. 3). The provisional generic formulation (see Fig. 2.1) should be used to aid the explanation, emphasizing that the goal of the treatment is to address the mechanisms maintaining binge eating and, if indicated, clinical obesity in an integrated and personalized way. Table 4.7 lists the points to cover when explaining CBT for BED to the patient.

Table 4.7 Points to be addressed when describing CBT for BED to patients

CBT for BED is one of the most promising treatments for people who have binge-eating episodes.
The treatment is adapted to the individual, and focuses primarily on what is acting to maintain a person's eating problems. It is, therefore, mainly focused on the present and the future, and addresses the problem's origins only if necessary.
The treatment will be tailored to their specific eating problem and needs, and will help them, with the aid of their therapist, to become an expert in their particular eating problems and the processes that maintain them.
Step One of the treatment (i.e., the first 4 weeks, 8 biweekly sessions), which includes two sessions a week, will be dedicated to improving their understanding of the psychological mechanisms that are maintaining their binge-eating episodes and, if indicated, clinical obesity. Other important goals of this step are reducing the frequency of binge-eating episodes and adopting an active lifestyle. In this part of the treatment, any attempt to lose weight is discouraged. Indeed, trying to lose weight before regularizing eating is like building a house without laying its foundations.
After 4 weeks, a Review Session will be dedicated to assessing the progress made, identifying any obstacles to change, and planning the next phase of treatment. From then on, the sessions will be held weekly.
Step Two of the treatment, will be personalized through the use of specific modules to address the psychological and behavioural mechanisms maintaining the BED and, if indicated, clinical obesity with cognitive behavioural strategies and procedures associated in some cases with the new weight-loss drugs (see Chap. 8). It lasts 20 weeks (8 weekly sessions plus 6 biweekly session), but in patients who achieve remission from eating-disorder psychopathology at the end of Step One and do not need to treat clinical obesity, it can be reduced to 3 sessions, 1 every 2 weeks.
Step Three of the treatment will be dedicated to preventing binge eating from recurring and maintaining a healthy weight. It lasts 12 weeks (3 sessions, 1 every 4 weeks), but in patients who addressed clinical obesity in Step Two, it lasts 48 weeks (12 sessions, 1 every 4 weeks).
If the patient gives consent, and agrees that it may be beneficial, significant others may be recruited to support a patient's efforts at changing their lifestyle and eating habits.
It is crucial that therapeutic momentum be maintained, and therefore that there are no interruptions in the treatment. Its success will depend on the therapist and patient working together, session by session, to tackle the mechanisms that maintain episodes of binge eating and excess weight.
Each appointment will last just under an hour, and the therapist must ensure that sessions start and end on time. It is advisable for the patient to arrive 15 minutes early so that they have time to prepare for the session.
The style of treatment is collaborative, and patients will be asked to play an active role, working together with their therapist as a team to overcome with their eating problem. To this end, they will agree from time to time on specific tasks to be carried out between sessions. These tasks are of paramount importance and must be given absolute priority. It is precisely what the patient does between encounters that will determine the limitations or benefits of the treatment.
The treatment should be considered a priority that requires commitment and a radical lifestyle change. The more effort the patient puts into the treatment, the more benefits they will attain.
Addressing the eating problem will be difficult, but worth it.

4.7 Actively Involving the Patient in the Decision to Change

As binge eating is associated with marked distress, guilt, and feelings of disgust with oneself [39], patients seeking treatment for BED are usually motivated to change, and appreciate the initial goal of CBT for BED to reduce the frequency of binge-eating episodes. However, they are often seeking a treatment that would resolve their eating problem without their active commitment (i.e., an external or "magic" solution). In such cases, the patient needs to be informed that, to resolve their eating problem effectively and for the long term, it is fundamental that they are actively involved in understanding the mechanisms maintaining their binge-eating episodes using real-time self-monitoring (see Chap. 5), and then to apply specific procedures agreed with the therapist to address the identified maintenance mechanisms.

Sometimes, it is more difficult to actively engage treatment-seeking patients whose primary goal is to lose weight. In such cases, it is advisable to discuss with the patient the pros and cons of focusing the first 4 weeks of the treatment (i.e., Step One) not on weight loss but only on understanding the mechanisms maintaining their binge-eating episodes, and then implementing specific procedures targeting said mechanisms with a view to reducing binge-eating frequency. Patients should be informed that weight loss will be addressed, but that the decision to do so will be made after 4 weeks, provided that there has been a marked reduction in binge-eating episodes. Indeed, if the binge eating continues, weight loss will be impossible to achieve, due to the mechanisms illustrated in the personal formulation. In patients who have previously tried to lose weight without addressing the mechanisms maintaining their binge-eating episodes, it is helpful to analyzse with them whether the persistence of binge-eating episodes had hampered their attempts. Most patients confirm that one of the most significant factors behind the failure of previous weight-loss attempts was, in fact, their binge-eating episodes, and they would therefore be open to addressing them.

Another essential aspect to consider before starting a patient on the programme is to assess whether they are ready. It is best not to begin CBT for BED until the odds of success are at their highest. So, if the patient has a holiday booked, or is about to get married, have a baby, start a new job or school, or move house etc., it is advisable to suggest they postpone the treatment until they can fully devote themselves to it. The patient must be free of commitments in the first 4 weeks of the treatment because a rapid response to treatment of BED, defined as a 70% reduction in binge-eating episodes after the first 4 weeks, predicts its long-term outcome [40].

Overcoming an eating disorder requires constant commitment, and it is therefore crucial that a patient be willing to make treatment an absolute priority. To ensure that this is the case, the therapist should ask the patient if they can put the programme at the forefront of their daily commitments. The therapist should tell the patient that planning meals and real-time self-monitoring will take 45–60 minutes a day. If they do not think they will be able to make the time for this, the therapist should help the patient make a list of their daily activities, and agree to put those that are not priorities to one side for the moment. In our experience, even the busiest people can devote 45–60 minutes daily to the programme. However, if a patient is adamant that they are unable to find the time, the therapist should still discuss the pros and cons of starting treatment, giving them an opportunity to re-assess their priorities. At the same time, the therapist should also try to help the patient in every practical way possible, scheduling appointment times to be compatible with their other commitments.

After having described the treatment (preferably with the aid of an information sheet) and allowing patients the opportunity to ask questions and express concerns, we suggest writing down the pros and cons of starting Step One of the treatment at home, and to bring a list of written questions to ask at the next appointment, which will focus on discussing these issues. This is especially important in ambivalent patients, for whom we schedule a second assessment and preparation session. In this session, we review the pros and cons of starting the treatment with the patient, seeking to reinforce interest in change and address any questions about CBT for BED. We also suggest that they "take the plunge" and try Step One of the programme as an experiment, repeating that the goal of this phase of the treatment is not weight loss but to have a better understanding of the psychological mechanisms that maintain their eating disorder and developing a regular pattern of eating. In patients who are very ambivalent about change, we schedule one additional session. However, this is not an expected outcome since most decide to start Step One of the programme after one or two sessions.

4.8 Coexisting Mental Disorders

CBT adopts a pragmatic approach to addressing mental disorders coexisting with BED [41]. In short, comorbidities should be recognized, but only assessed for treatment when significant and having clinical implications. Hence, we find it clinically useful to divide comorbidity into three main groups [41]:

1. *Disorders that do not interfere with CBT for BED and that will probably respond to it.* These disorders should be recognized, monitored, and re-assessed during treatment, but need not be focused on specifically. Examples are:
   - Secondary depression (attributable to the eating disorder)
   - Social anxiety (attributable to the eating disorder)
2. *Disorders that do not respond to CBT for BED but do not interfere with the treatment.* These disorders must be recognized, and a decision must be made on when to address them. As a general rule, it is advisable to treat such disorders either before or after tackling the eating-disorder psychopathology, especially if they need to be managed via psychological treatments. Examples are as follows:
   - Post-traumatic stress disorder, including reported sexual abuse
   - Obsessive-compulsive disorder (which may be treated using selective serotonin reuptake inhibitors (SSRIs) during treatment for the eating disorder)
3. *Disorders that interfere with the treatment of BED.* These disorders need to be recognized and addressed before starting CBT. Examples are as follows:
   - Continuous substance misuse

- Acute psychotic disorders
- Acute type 1 or type 2 bipolar disorder
- Clinical depression (not attributable to eating disorder)

Below are described the strategies we use for the management of clinical depression and anxiety disorders, the two psychiatric disorders that most frequently coexist with BED [42].

4.8.1 Clinical Depression

Coexisting mood disorders have been reported in more than 50% of patients with BED [43]. However, a diagnosis of coexisting clinical depression, also known as major depression or major depressive disorder, is often inappropriate. This is because there is a substantial conceptual overlap between some features of the two disorders. Indeed, many features used in the diagnosis of clinical depression are known to be the consequence of recurrent binge-eating episodes [43]. Examples are as follows: self-criticism, low mood, social withdrawal, shame, guilt, and feelings of impotence. In addition, patients with BED often report the absence of these features on the days when they do not binge. Changes in mood secondary to the clinical features of BED regress with remission of the disorder and therefore do not need to be addressed directly.

To prevent the superfluous prescription of antidepressants, it is important to discern whether the coexistence of BED and depression constitutes a true or spurious comorbidity. Truly coexisting clinical depression hinders the treatment of the eating disorder and must therefore be identified and treated. Indeed, those suffering from coexisting clinical depression think that change will be impossible and will not have sufficient energy to engage in treatment, nor enough concentration to understand and retain the information provided. Features suggestive that clinical depression is concomitant with BED are the following: a personal history of clinical depression before the onset of the eating disorder, late eating-disorder onset, recent intensification of depressive features in the absence of any change in the eating-disorder psychopathology (e.g., low mood, social withdrawal, or suicidal thoughts and plans), loss of interest, crying, recurrent thoughts on the pointlessness of life, personal neglect. The more of these features that the patient reports, the more confident we are that a separate diagnosis of clinical depression is warranted.

In patients seeking treatment for BED with coexisting clinical depression, it is advisable to prescribe antidepressant medications (e.g., fluoxetine or sertraline) at full dosage for 9 months. The choice to use medication and not psychotherapy for the treatment of clinical depression depends on two observations [44]: (i) psychotherapy is time-consuming, and its progress will in any event be hampered by the eating disorder, and (ii) antidepressant medications generally work well. However, some patients have reservations about taking antidepressants, but these typically depend on clinical depression itself. In such cases, a patient's reluctance should be explored by providing the following information:

- Taking antidepressants is not a sign of weakness.
- Antidepressants do not interfere with one's ability to do things in life.
- Antidepressants are non-addictive, do not affect mood (they only treat depression) and have few side effects.
- Taken for less than 1 year, fluoxetine and sertraline do not increase appetite or weight. There is only an increased sensitivity to the intoxicating effects of alcohol, so one has to drink with caution.
- The resolution of clinical depression allows for effective psychotherapy for eating disorders.
- Fluoxetine may directly result in a decreased frequency of binge-eating episodes and some secondary clinical features of BED (fear of losing control, secondary depression, but only rarely concern about weight and body shape). This effect has also been observed in patients without depression.

4.8.2 Anxiety Disorders

Anxiety disorders are present in about 30% of patients with BED [43]. However, unlike coexisting clinical depression, an anxiety disorder, although frequent, does not pose major problems as regards patient management. Note though, that when the features of an anxiety disorder coexist with clinical depression, they may be secondary to it. In this case, we recommend treating the anxiety through the depression, as per the indications above.

The first question we ask ourselves when evaluating patients is whether the features of the anxiety disorder co-exist with or are secondary to BED. Some examples of anxiety disorder features that stem from the eating disorder are avoiding socializing due to difficulties eating in front of others or avoiding being seen or exposing one's body. These characteristics are not indicative of social phobia because the fear is attributable to the psychopathology of the eating disorder.

The second question we ask is whether the features of the coexisting anxiety disorder could interfere with the treatment. If the anxiety disorder is truly comorbid, this is likely to be the case. For example, a person with agoraphobia may have a lot of difficulty making some of the changes required by CBT for BED, for example, exposing their body in social situations, eating in public, and, in severe cases, even attending sessions. It is obvious that in such cases, the agoraphobia must be resolved before the patient begins treatment for their eating disorder.

The third question we ask ourselves is whether the features of the anxiety disorder are likely to resolve with remission from BED. In our clinical experience, this is frequently the case, and for this reason, if the anxiety disorder does not represent an insurmountable barrier to treatment, we do not address it directly, and we proceed directly to CBT for BED.

References

1. Lydecker JA, Galbraith K, Ivezaj V, White MA, Barnes RD, Roberto CA, et al. Words will never hurt me? Preferred terms for describing obesity and binge eating. Int J Clin Pract. 2016;70(8):682–90. https://doi.org/10.1111/ijcp.12835.
2. Coffino JA, Udo T, Grilo CM. Rates of help-seeking in US adults with lifetime DSM-5 eating disorders: prevalence across diagnoses and differences by sex and ethnicity/race. Mayo Clin Proc. 2019;94(8):1415–26. https://doi.org/10.1016/j.mayocp.2019.02.030.
3. Cossrow N, Pawaskar M, Witt EA, Ming EE, Victor TW, Herman BK, et al. Estimating the prevalence of binge eating disorder in a community sample from the United States: comparing DSM-IV-TR and DSM-5 criteria. J Clin Psychiatry. 2016;77(8):e968–74. https://doi.org/10.4088/JCP.15m10059.
4. Supina D, Herman BK, Frye CB, Shillington AC. Knowledge of binge eating disorder: a cross-sectional survey of physicians in the United States. Postgrad Med. 2016;128(3):311–6. https://doi.org/10.1080/00325481.2016.1157441.
5. Lean ME, Han TS, Morrison CE. Waist circumference as a measure for indicating need for weight management. BMJ. 1995;311(6998):158–61. https://doi.org/10.1136/bmj.311.6998.158.
6. Chan JM, Rimm EB, Colditz GA, Stampfer MJ, Willett WC. Obesity, fat distribution, and weight gain as risk factors for clinical diabetes in men. Diabetes Care. 1994;17(9):961–9. https://doi.org/10.2337/diacare.17.9.961.
7. Dalle Grave R, Sartirana M, El Ghoch M, Calugi S. Treating obesity with personalized cognitive behavioral therapy. Cham: Springer; 2018.
8. Wilson GT, Fairburn CC, Agras WS, Walsh BT, Kraemer H. Cognitive-behavioral therapy for bulimia nervosa: time course and mechanisms of change. J Consult Clin Psychol. 2002;70(2):267–74. https://doi.org/10.1037/0022-006X.70.2.267.
9. Kushner RF. Clinical assessment of patients with obesity. In: Brownell KD, Walsh BT, editors. Eating disorders and obesity. New York: Guilford Press; 2017. p. 473–9.
10. Wharton S, Raiber L, Serodio KJ, Lee J, Christensen RA. Medications that cause weight gain and alternatives in Canada: a narrative review. Diabetes Metab Syndr Obes. 2018;11:427–38. https://doi.org/10.2147/DMSO.S171365.
11. Calugi S, Milanese C, Sartirana M, El Ghoch M, Sartori F, Geccherle E, et al. The Eating Disorder Examination Questionnaire: reliability and validity of the Italian version. Eat Weight Disord. 2017;22(3):509–14. https://doi.org/10.1007/s40519-016-0276-6.
12. Fairburn CG, Cooper Z, O'Connor M. Eating Disorder Examination Questionnaire (EDE-Q 6.0). In: Fairburn CG, editor. Cognitive behavior therapy and eating disorders. New York: Guilford Press; 2008. p. 309–13.
13. Calugi S, Sartirana M, Milanese C, El Ghoch M, Riolfi F, Dalle GR. The clinical impairment assessment questionnaire: validation in Italian patients with eating disorders. Eat Weight Disord. 2018;23(5):685–94. https://doi.org/10.1007/s40519-018-0477-2
14. Bohn K, Doll HA, Cooper Z, O'Connor M, Palmer RL, Fairburn CG. The measurement of impairment due to eating disorder psychopathology. Behav Res Ther. 2008;46(10):1105–10. https://doi.org/10.1016/j.brat.2008.06.012.
15. Derogatis LR, Spencer MS. The Brief Symptom Inventory (BSI): administration, scoring, and procedures manual-I. Baltimore: Johns Hopkins University School of Medicine, Clinical Psychometrics Research Unit; 1982.
16. Dalle Grave R, Soave F, Ruocco A, Dametti L, Calugi S. Quality of life and physical performance in patients with obesity: a network analysis. Nutrients. 2020;12(3):602. https://doi.org/10.3390/nu12030602.
17. McHorney CA, Ware JE Jr, Raczek AE. The MOS 36-Item Short-Form Health Survey (SF-36): II. Psychometric and clinical tests of validity in measuring physical and mental health constructs. Med Care. 1993;31(3):247–63. https://doi.org/10.1097/00005650-199303000-00006.

18. Innamorati M, Imperatori C, Lamis DA, Contardi A, Castelnuovo G, Tamburello S, et al. Weight Bias Internalization scale discriminates obese and overweight patients with different severity levels of depression: The Italian version of the WBIS. Curr Psychol. 2017;36:242–51.
19. Durso LE, Latner JD. Understanding self-directed stigma: development of the weight bias internalization scale. Obesity. 2008;16(Suppl 2):S80–6. https://doi.org/10.1038/oby.2008.448.
20. Calugi S, Ricca V, Castellini G, Lo Sauro C, Ruocco A, Chignola E, et al. The Eating Disorder Examination: reliability and validity of the Italian version. Eat Weight Disord. 2015;20(4):505–11. https://doi.org/10.1007/s40519-015-0191-2.
21. Fairburn CG, Cooper Z, O'Connor M. Eating Disorder Examination. In: Fairburn CG, editor. Cognitive behavior therapy and eating disorders. New York: Guilford Press; 2008. p. 265–308.
22. Fairburn C, Cooper Z. The Eating Disorder Examination. In: Fairburn C, Wilson G, editors. Binge eating: nature, assessment, and treatment. New York: Guilford Press; 1993. p. 317–60.
23. Bray GA, Kim KK, Wilding JPH. Obesity: a chronic relapsing progressive disease process. A position statement of the World Obesity Federation. Obes Rev. 2017;18(7):715–23. https://doi.org/10.1111/obr.12551.
24. Wharton S, Lau DCW, Vallis M, Sharma AM, Biertho L, Campbell-Scherer D, et al. Obesity in adults: a clinical practice guideline. CMAJ. 2020;192(31):E875–E91. https://doi.org/10.1503/cmaj.191707.
25. Blüher M. Metabolically healthy obesity. Endocr Rev. 2020;41:3. https://doi.org/10.1210/endrev/bnaa004.
26. Zembic A, Eckel N, Stefan N, Baudry J, Schulze MB. An empirically derived definition of metabolically healthy obesity based on risk of cardiovascular and total mortality. JAMA Netw Open. 2021;4(5):e218505. https://doi.org/10.1001/jamanetworkopen.2021.8505.
27. Dalle Grave R. New Obesity framework: overcoming stigma and improving care; we need a shared definition of the diagnosis of clinical obesity. Posted October 20, 2023. Psychol Today. 2023.
28. Rubino F, Batterham RL, Koch M, Mingrone G, le Roux CW, Farooqi IS, et al. Lancet diabetes & endocrinology commission on the definition and diagnosis of clinical obesity. Lancet Diabetes Endocrinol. 2023;11(4):226–8. https://doi.org/10.1016/S2213-8587(23)00058-X.
29. Dalle Grave R, Sartirana M, El Ghoch M, Calugi S. Trattare l'obesità con la terapia cognitivo comportamentale personalizzata. Verona: Positive Press; 2019.
30. Meichenbaum D, Gilmore JRI. Resistance: from a cognitive–behavioral perspective. In: Wachtel P, editor. Resistance: psychodynamic and behavioral approaches. New York: Plenum; 1982. p. 133–56.
31. Guidano VF, Liotti G. Cognitive processes and emotional disorders: a structural approach to psychotherapy. New York: Guilford Press; 1983.
32. Linehan MM. Cognitive-behavioral treatment of borderline personality disorder. New York: Guilford Press; 1993.
33. Miller WR, Rollnick S. Motivational interviewing. 2nd ed. New York: Guilford Press; 2002.
34. Bandura A. Social foundations of thought and action: a social cognitive theory. Englewood Cliffs: Prentice-Hall; 1986.
35. Strecher VJ, DeVellis BM, Becker MH, Rosenstock IM. The role of self-efficacy in achieving health behavior change. Health Educ Q. 1986;13(1):73–92. https://doi.org/10.1177/109019818601300108.
36. Ciao AC, Latner JD, Durso LE. Treatment seeking and barriers to weight loss treatments of different intensity levels among obese and overweight individuals. Eat Weight Disord. 2012;17(1):e9–16. https://doi.org/10.1007/bf03325323.
37. Reddon H, Gueant JL, Meyre D. The importance of gene-environment interactions in human obesity. Clin Sci (Lond). 2016;130(18):1571–97. https://doi.org/10.1042/cs20160221.
38. Jensen MD, Ryan DH, Apovian CM, Ard JD, Comuzzie AG, Donato KA, et al. AHA/ACC/TOS guideline for the management of overweight and obesity in adults: a report of the American College of Cardiology/American Heart Association Task Force on Practice Guidelines and The Obesity Society. J Am Coll Cardiol. 2013;63(25 Pt B):2985–3023. https://doi.org/10.1016/j.jacc.2013.11.004.

39. American Psychiatric Association. Diagnostic and statistical manual of mental disorders, (DSM-5). Arlington: American Psychiatric Publishing; 2013.
40. Grilo CM, White MA, Wilson GT, Gueorguieva R, Masheb RM. Rapid response predicts 12-month post-treatment outcomes in binge-eating disorder: theoretical and clinical implications. Psychol Med. 2012;42(4):807–17. https://doi.org/10.1017/s0033291711001875.
41. Dalle Grave R, Sartirana M, Calugi S. Complex cases and comorbidity in eating disorders. Assessment and management. Cham: Springer Nature; 2021.
42. Citrome L. Binge-eating disorder and comorbid conditions: differential diagnosis and implications for treatment. J Clin Psychiatry. 2017;78(Suppl 1):9–13. https://doi.org/10.4088/JCP.sh16003su1c.02.
43. Grilo CM, White MA, Masheb RM. DSM-IV psychiatric disorder comorbidity and its correlates in binge eating disorder. Int J Eat Disord. 2009;42(3):228–34. https://doi.org/10.1002/eat.20599.
44. Dalle Grave R, Sartirana M, Calugi S. La gestione dei casi complessi nei disturbi dell'alimentazione. Verona: Positive Press; 2019.

Part II

The Core Protocol

The Three Steps of CBT for BED

5

Abstract

CBT for BED is organized into three steps. Step One lasts 4 weeks, involves two sessions per week, and has the goals of increasing the patient's understanding of the cognitive behavioural mechanisms that maintain BED, reducing weight concerns and the frequency of binge-eating episodes, and adopting an active lifestyle. A Review Session is planned at the end of Step One to review progress made over the first 4 weeks, as well as to identify any obstacles and plan the next treatment step. Step Two lasts about 20 weeks and involves one session weekly for the first 2 months and then one session every 2 weeks. However, in patients who achieve complete remission of their eating-disorder psychopathology early, and do not need or wish to address weight loss, the duration of Step Two can be reduced to three to four biweekly sessions. In this step, the procedures begun in Step One continue to be applied, and the treatment is personalized with specific modules to address the eating-disorder psychopathology operating in the individual patient and, if indicated, achieve and accept reasonable and healthy weight loss. Step Three lasts 48 weeks and involves one session every 4 weeks. However, in patients in whom weight loss was not addressed during Step Two, the duration of Step Three can be reduced to two to three sessions. The goals of this step are to prevent binge eating from recurring and to ensure a healthy weight is maintained.

5.1 Step One: Starting Well

The degree of change achieved in the first 4 weeks of treatment of BED is a strong predictor of outcome [1]. For this reason, it is fundamental to start the treatment well. The patient and the therapist must be ready to begin, and any potential impediments to treatment must be addressed in Session 0 (see Chap. 6).

R. Dalle Grave et al., *Cognitive Behavior Therapy for Binge Eating Disorder*,
https://doi.org/10.1007/978-3-031-71456-6_5

5.1.1 Goals

Step One has five main goals:

1. To engage the patient in the treatment and change
2. To create an individualized personal formulation to guide the treatment
3. To provide psychoeducation and reduce concerns about weight
4. To establish a pattern of regular eating
5. To develop an active lifestyle

5.1.2 Structure

The structure of Step One is relatively standard because the procedures are introduced in a precise, sequential fashion, albeit on a personalized basis. Step One lasts 4 weeks, and the patient is seen for two 50-minute weekly sessions.

5.1.3 Content

The top priority is actively engaging the patient in the treatment and the need to make changes. Indeed, CBT for BED has little chance of success unless the patient is fully engaged. Therefore, the therapist should become skilled at engaging patients in both the process of change and the treatment itself. This task is one of the most important challenges because, even if many patients agree on most aspects of the treatment (e.g., addressing binge-eating episodes and clinical obesity), there are other elements that they may find problematic (e.g., seeing the treatment as a priority, playing an active role in the treatment).

After having engaged the patients, the next goal is to address the clinical features that are playing an influential role in maintaining the individual's eating-disorder psychopathology. To this end, we generally compare the psychopathology of eating disorders to a house of cards [2], which can easily be collapsed by removing the cards at the bottom. This analogy helps explain why the treatment does not need to address every clinical feature the patient presents. Indeed, many clinical features (e.g., concerns about eating, shape and weight) disappear once the key clinical features reinforcing them have been removed. So, a crucial task of the therapist is to work together with the patient to identify and address the key clinical features that are maintaining their manifestation of BED. This can be achieved through the provision of personalized education on the patient's eating disorder by drafting a personal formulation. This will help elucidate the main mechanisms maintaining their eating problems, and will be a stepping stone to diminishing their concerns about weight and establishing a pattern of regular eating, which is considered one of the most potent procedures for reducing the frequency of binge-eating episodes [2].

With adolescent patients, parents are always involved in their child's treatment. Their role is, however, as "helpers", assisting the patient achieve change and

Table 5.1 Step One: main procedures and general timeframe

Week number	1		2		3		4	
Session number	0	1	2	3	4	5	6	7
Assessment	√	(√)						
Creating the formulation	√	(√)						
Self-monitoring	√	√	√	√	√	√	√	√
Collaborative weighing		√		√		√		√
EPCL-BED		√		√		√		√
Adopting an active lifestyle		√	√	√	√	√	√	√
Regular eating			√	√	√	√	√	√
Psychoeducation	√	√	√	√	√	√	√	√
Involving significant others		√[a]	√		√			√

EPCL eating problem checklist, *BED* binge-eating disorder
[a]In adolescent patients: session with parents alone between Sessions 0 and 1

creating an optimum family environment, rather than "controllers". With the patient's prior consent, they may also be recruited to help implement certain treatment procedures [3]. Parental involvement is generally managed through one session with parents alone in the first week of treatment, and then several joint sessions of about 15 minutes with the adolescent and the therapist together at the end of sessions with the patient alone (see also Chap. 10). Significant others may also provide assistance to adult patients, and if the latter agree, may participate in joint sessions held at the end individual sessions.

Table 5.1 shows the main procedures of Step One and the appropriate timeframe for their implementation.

5.1.4 Desirable Outcome

At the end of Step One, the therapist should have developed a solid collaborative relationship with the patient and have a good understanding of their eating disorder and individual circumstances. The patients should have become fully engaged in the treatment and change, and reached an understanding of their eating disorder and the main processes maintaining it (as a result of their personal formulation and real-time self-monitoring). They should have become less concerned about their weight (as a result of collaborative weighing), implemented a stable and regular pattern of eating, and reduced the frequency of binge eating (as a result of regular eating), and, if applicable, increased the number of daily steps.

Adverse outcomes at this stage are infrequent, but include interrupting the treatment, disliking CBT, or failing to implement or adhere to self-monitoring and/or collaborative weighing procedures. Other patients may have difficulties in complying with regular eating or have a comorbidity or circumstance (e.g., coexisting clinical depression) that is interfering with their progress. If it is not possible to effectively address the obstacles to these issues, the therapist should recommend another type of treatment.

5.2 Review Session: Taking Stock

A review session is introduced after the end of Step One in all patients, with a view to delivering a treatment that is both flexible and highly individualized. This session should be dedicated to reviewing the patient's progress, identifying any emerging barriers to change, modifying the personal formulation as needed, and planning Step Two of the treatment, which may or may not include the goal of achieving healthy weight loss. It is essential that this review session be used to identify patients who are not doing well, because they are unlikely to achieve a good outcome unless the reasons for their poor response are not recognized and addressed.

5.3 Step Two: Addressing the Change

This is the main body of CBT for BED. It has the aim of addressing both the main mechanisms that are maintaining the patient's eating-disorder psychopathology, and helping patients to reach a reasonable and healthy weight loss, where appropriate. How this is achieved will vary from patient to patient.

5.3.1 Goals

Step Two has three main goals:

1. To address the remaining eating-disorder features, including weight loss (if indicated)
2. To disrupt the mechanisms maintaining the individual's eating-disorder psychopathology
3. To develop skills for tackling setbacks

5.3.2 Structure

In Step Two, the treatment becomes highly personalized, being tailored to the patient's individual psychopathology. Patients are seen once a week for the first 2 months, and subsequently every 2 weeks. All Step Two content, strategies, and procedures are to be dictated by patient-specific problems. Any involvement of significant others should be flexible and appropriate, and be managed as described in Step One.

5.3.3 Content

Step Two addresses the remaining eating-disorder features by continuing to implement the strategies and procedures introduced in Step One (i.e., weekly weighing, regular eating) and introducing others. The aim is to disrupt the maintenance mechanisms at play with a view to obtaining remission from eating disorder, and a healthy level of weight loss if indicated. To achieve these goals, one or more of the following modules should be used, as appropriate (covered in detail in Chaps. 12, 13, 14, 15, 16, 17, 18 and 19):

- Healthy Weight Loss
- Events, Moods, and Eating
- Dysfunctional Dieting
- Overvaluation of Shape and Weight
- Unrealistic Weight Goals
- Internalized Weight Stigma
- Setbacks and Mindsets
- Maintenance Preparation

The decision about which modules to use and the order in which to employ them should be based primarily on their relative contribution to the eating-disorder psychopathology in the individual patient. Then the time likely required to complete them should be weighed against the need for early progress. Towards the end of Step Two, the Setbacks and Mindsets and Maintenance Preparation modules should be introduced. This will lay the ground for further work on staying well in the future, the focus in Step Three of treatment.

In patients who achieve complete remission of binge-eating episodes, do not display any other eating-disorder psychopathology (as confirmed by the EDE-Q), and do not need to address clinical obesity (see Sect. 4.3.1 and Table 4.4 for the definition) after the end of Step One, Step Two only need implement the Setbacks and Mindsets and Maintenance Preparation modules, and be delivered across three biweekly sessions.

Figure 5.1 shows the Step Two modules and the indications on which to use.

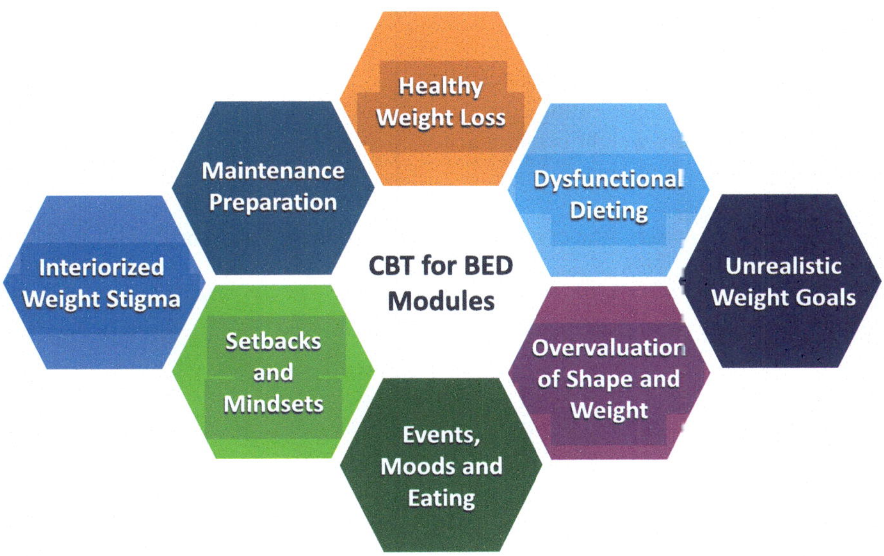

Fig. 5.1 The modules of CBT for BED

5.4 Step Three: Preventing Relapse

Step Three is the last part of the treatment and is aimed at preventing binge eating from recurring, maintaining a healthy weight, and ending the treatment well. Indeed, it is just as crucial that the treatment end as begin well.

5.4.1 Goals

Step Three has four main goals:

1. Minimizing the risk of binge-eating relapse
2. Maintaining a healthy weight
3. Addressing patients' concerns about ending treatment
4. Phasing out specific treatment procedures

5.4.2 Structure

Step Three involves one session every 4 weeks and lasts 48 weeks. However, in patients who have addressed clinical obesity with the Healthy Weight Loss module in Step Two, it is extended to 12 sessions, 1 very 4 weeks. The usual structure is retained throughout, but the sessions are focused on preventing relapse.

5.4.3 Content

Step Three has four components:

1. Using and refining the maintenance plan
2. Making sure any binge-eating episode does not become a relapse
3. Ensuring a healthy weight is maintained
4. Winding up the treatment

Figure 5.2 summarizes the content of the three steps of CBT for BED.

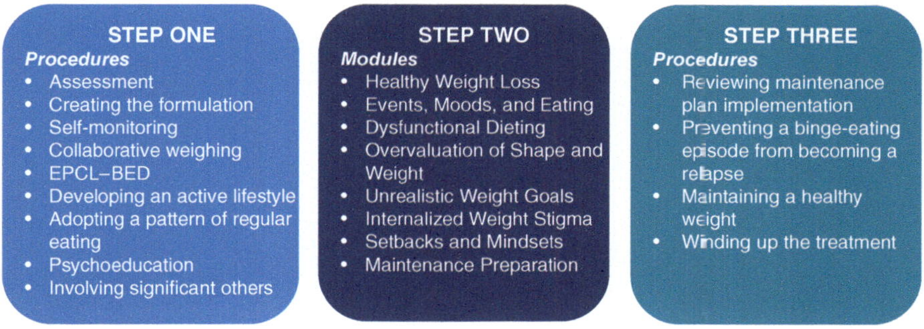

Fig. 5.2 The main procedures of the three steps of CBT for BED

References

1. Grilo CM, White MA, Wilson GT, Gueorguieva R, Masheb RM. Rapid response predicts 12-month post-treatment outcomes in binge-eating disorder: theoretical and clinical implications. Psychol Med. 2012;42(4):807–17. https://doi.org/10.1017/s0033291711001875.
2. Fairburn CG. Cognitive behavior therapy and eating disorders. New York: Guilford Press; 2008.
3. Dalle Grave R, el Khazen C. Cognitive behaviour therapy for eating disorders in young people: a parents' guide. London: Routledge; 2022.

Session 0

6

Abstract

We call the first session of cognitive behaviour therapy (CBT) for binge-eating disorder (BED) Session 0 because it represents the baseline, or starting point. It includes five components, the first of which is engaging the patient in treatment and the process of change. To this end, the therapist needs to pay careful attention to their attitude toward the patient and the words used to address the topics of binge eating and clinical obesity, and avoid any verbal or non-verbal expressions of weight stigma. The second component is assessing the current state of the patient's eating disorder, with reference to the previous 4 weeks. The third component is collaboratively creating the personal formulation, a visual representation (a flow chart) of the processes that appear to be maintaining the patient's binge-eating episodes and, if present, clinical obesity. The fourth component is informing the patient about the nature of the treatment. The fifth and last component is introducing real-time self-monitoring, a key procedure of CBT for BED that consists of self-reporting, on a dedicated monitoring record, the relevant behaviours, thoughts, emotions, and events "in the moment" in which they are experienced. Finally, the session is concluded by summarizing its content, restating the homework assignment(s), and scheduling the next appointment.

Session 0 has a relatively fixed content that encompasses the following five "tasks":

1. Engaging the patient in treatment and change
2. Assessing the problem
3. Creating the formulation
4. Informing the patient about the treatment
5. Introducing real-time self-monitoring

R. Dalle Grave et al., *Cognitive Behavior Therapy for Binge Eating Disorder*, https://doi.org/10.1007/978-3-031-71456-6_6

6.1 Engaging the Patient in Treatment and Change

If Session 0 is delivered by a therapist other than the one who conducted the assessment and preparation for CBT, the therapist must be aware that the patient will be sizing them up in the same way that they will be assessing the patient. For this reason, the therapist needs to be scrupulously attentive to their attitude towards them. They must carefully choose the words they use to address the topics of binge eating and clinical obesity (see Sect. 4.3.1 and Table 4.4 for the definition), and avoid any verbal or non-verbal expressions of weight stigma.

The general guidelines suggested by CBT for BED on how to become an engaging therapist have already been described in the Assessment, Preparation and Medical Management phase (see Chap. 4). These should also be adhered to in Session 0 and throughout the course of treatment. Our clinical experience practicing CBT for BED has led us to conclude that engaging the patient does not take much motivational work as the treatment has been designed to be intrinsically motivating. Note, however, that the factor most favourable to patient engagement is likely to hinge on the therapist's behaviour. Previous patients have reported that they particularly appreciate feeling being heard and understood, not stigmatized for their weight. The rapid reduction of binge-eating episodes they achieve over the early sessions also provides a powerful boost to their motivation.

6.2 Assessing the Problem

The main objective in Session 0 is to re-assess the current state of the patient's eating disorder (see "Current status" in Table 4.1 of Chap. 4) by referring to the preceding 4 weeks (28 days). Careful and detailed attention should be paid to the processes that are acting to maintain the patient's eating disorder (diagnosed in the Assessment and Preparation phase), which should be recorded on the patient's initial personal formulation. Take care not to overlook features secondary to binge-eating episodes and clinical obesity, or the presence of internalized weight stigma, or their respective effects on physical health and psychosocial functioning. This is an opportunity to get a full clinical picture of the patient's individual problems, which will dictate how the treatment will unfold.

6.3 Creating the Formulation

6.3.1 What Is a Formulation?

The personal formulation is a visual representation (a flow chart) of the processes that appear to be maintaining the patient's binge-eating episodes and, if present, clinical obesity [1].

6.3.2 Purpose

The personal formulation is created for the following reasons [2, 3]:

- It promotes patient engagement in the treatment because it helps them to understand their eating- and weight-related problems.
- It helps the patient understand the self-perpetuating nature of their problems (i.e., being trapped in a series of mutually reinforcing maintenance mechanisms): a piece of information generally appreciated by the patient because it explains why they find it difficult to enact change.
- It helps the patient to distance themselves from their problem, to take a step back, to take a "decentred" position by piquing their interest and intriguing them in their eating disorder and the processes that are maintaining it.
- It helps the patient and the therapist to identify the targets of the treatment (as such it is a "road map" for the programme), and to understand which features of their problem and maintenance mechanisms to address and in what order.
- It makes the patient feel in control because it promotes an understanding of what will need to be addressed by the treatment.

It is important to emphasize that the personal formulation is not a visual representation of the hypothetical processes that may have favoured the *onset* of the eating disorder and clinical obesity. If the patient is perplexed by the fact that treatment does not address the origins of their problems, they should be informed that the cause of BED is not yet understood, and that studies show that it is possible to achieve remission from an eating disorder without understanding the root cause. That being said, we do reassure patients that they will have an opportunity to discuss the inception of their issues later on, when the principal processes that are maintaining the eating disorder have been interrupted.

6.3.3 How to Create a Formulation

Figure 2.1, which shows a composite transdiagnostic formulation of the main factors maintaining binge-eating episodes in people with BED, can be used as a model to create the patient's individual formulation. The more familiar the therapist becomes with this model, the easier it will be for them to create a formulation that adapts to the psychopathology operating in each patient.

Creating the personal formulation must be done well, and it is a skill that develops with practice. It should be drawn slowly, step by step, and legibly on an A4 sheet of paper, placed between the therapist and the patient, who should be seated so that they can clearly see what the therapist is doing (e.g., at the corner of the desk). The therapist's role is to guide its construction while taking care to keep the patient engaged.

The personal formulation should include only the main processes that seem to have operated to maintain the binge-eating episodes over the last 28 days. Avoid including too many things so as not to confuse the patient. However, it should be emphasized that this formulation is a provisional iteration and will have to be modified during the course of treatment, as new information emerges.

It is best to start the personal formulation by focusing on something that the patient expressly wants to change (e.g., binge-eating episodes or clinical obesity). If appropriate, the patient's own terms should be used in this discussion, which should unfold as in the following example transcript illustrating the creation of a personal formulation with a patient with BED and clinical obesity.

Therapist: Thank you for the information you have shared with me. Now, I would like us to analyse the main factors that appear to be fuelling your eating problem. If you agree, we'll start by drawing on this sheet of paper what I have understood about your problem (*the therapist holds a blank A4 sheet of paper between themself and the patient*).

Patient: I agree.

Therapist: Please tell me if you agree or disagree with anything I write, and let me know if something in my explanation is unclear to you or does not add up.

Patient: Okay.

Therapist: Well, If I have understood correctly, you are feeling very down because you think that your eating and weight are out of your control.

Patient: Yes, that's right. I feel sad and guilty because I binge, eat too much, and snack too often during the day.

Therapist: Okay, then we could start by including binge-eating, and what we call "overeating" and uncontrolled, or "dysregulated", eating. Do you understand (*the therapist writes* "binge-eating, overeating, and dysregulated eating" *in the centre of the sheet*)?

Patient: Yes.

Therapist: It seems to me that these episodes make you feel very, very bad... Why do you think that is?

Patient: Er... because by eating in this way, I am putting on more and more weight, and I am already suffering from prediabetes, hypertension and knee arthritis. My doctor says I have clinical obesity. I am very unhappy with my shape and weight.

Therapist: (*The therapist writes* "clinical obesity" and next to "binge-eating episodes, overeating, and dysregulated eating" and *connects them with two bidirectional arrows*). So, you are concerned about the effect of weight on your health, dissatisfied with your shape and weight, and this makes you feel sad and guilty?

Patient: Yes, very much so.

Therapist: (*The therapist writes* "concerns about the effects of weight on health, and body dissatisfaction" and "clinical obesity" above and next to them, respectively, and *draws arrows to show how they are connected to* "binge-eating episodes, overeating, and dysregulated eating. And what do you do to manage these concerns after a binge-eating episode?

Patient: Sometimes nothing, but occasionally, I skip a meal or have a day or two where I try to cut out carbs to lose weight, even though I often can't.

Therapist: So you skip meals and cut out carbs after you eat too much or binge because you are worried about your weight and dissatisfied with your body (*The therapist makes the entry* "skipping meals and cutting out carbs", and *draws arrows to it from* "binge-eating episodes and overeating and dysregulated eating" *and* "concerns about the effects of gaining weight on health, and body dissatisfaction")?

Patient: (*Looking at the diagram*) Yes, that's right!

Therapist: Would I be correct in saying that your attempts to restrict eating are then interrupted by a new binge-eating episode (*the therapist draws an arrow from* "skipping meals and avoiding carbs" *to* "binge-eating episode")?

Patient: Yes, that's right.

Therapist: Alright. You should know that this typically occurs through two mechanisms. The first arises when you attempt to cut back on your food by imposing what we call "extreme and rigid dietary rules" in response to a binge-eating episode or in the attempt to lose weight (*the therapist draws arrows from* "clinical obesity" *and* "binge-eating episode" *to* "skipping meals and avoiding carbs"), when you are concerned about the effects of gaining weight on your health and experiencing body dissatisfaction. We call dietary rules "extreme" when there are a lot of them and they are very difficult to follow. This means they are very easy to break, especially when you are distracted or feeling strong emotions. We call dietary rules "rigid" when you interpret even the slightest deviation from them as a total loss of control. Would that be fair to say?

Patient: Yes, that sounds right.

Therapist: This can be described as "all-or-nothing" thinking. You feel you are losing control, so you might as well give up.

Patient: That sounds familiar.

Therapist: And would I be right in saying that in this frame of mind you are more susceptible to a binge-eating episode?

Patient: Yes. That's exactly what happens to me.

Therapist: Also, you told me that as you have put on weight, you have developed arthritis of the knee. Has this changed your activity levels in any way?

Patient: Yes. I was never into sports, but before my knee problems, I used to walk more and go to the gym at least once a week.

Therapist: Did you stop going to the gym because of your knee problems?

Patient: Yes. But also because I am ashamed to be seen doing physical activity with this fat body.

Therapist: So, if I understand you correctly, a sedentary lifestyle has partially contributed to your weight gain (the therapist makes the entry "sedentary lifestyle", and draws an arrow from it to "clinical obesity"), but also that your clinical obesity has contributed to your sedentary lifestyle (*the therapist draws an arrow from* "clinical obesity" to "sedentary lifestyle").

Patient: Yes. That's just the way it is.

Therapist: Right. One more question. You told me that your higher weight makes you ashamed to go to the gym. How so?

Patient: People would think I am ridiculous. Too fat to exercise. And they would be right. I look disgusting, and it is my fault because I am weak and have no willpower.

Therapist: I am sorry you think this way about yourself. However, scientific research tells us that binge eating is not merely a matter of willpower. It is a psychological problem propped up by several maintenance processes. A kind of vicious cycle. Do you see (*indicating the formulation*)?

Patient: Yes. That's good to know!

Therapist: At the same time, your weight is determined by several genetic and environmental factors that alter your body's regulation of hunger and satiety (*drawing an arrow from* "clinical obesity" *to* "binge eating episodes, overeating and dysregulated eating"). It seems to me that you have come to believe that you overeat because you are lazy, weak or greedy.

Patient: I think you are right. When I was skinny, I felt fine. Now I'm heavier, I often feel down, and unable to control my eating and weight.

Therapist: This indicates to me that you have what we call "internalized social weight stigma", when a person applies negative societal or cultural beliefs about body weight to themselves. Know, however, that several scientific studies have shown that internalized weight stigma can be linked to negative body image, depression and lack of self-efficacy—the feeling that you are unable to change your eating, overeating, binge eating and low level of physical activity. Internalized weight stigma is a problem that we will have to deal with, as are your negative emotions, such as guilt and sadness (*the therapist makes the entries* "interiorized weight stigma" *and* "guilt and sadness" *and draws arrows to them from* "clinical obesity"). Is it true that you often overeat or binge when you feel down?

Patient: Yes. That is exactly the case.

Therapist: (*draws arrows from* "guilt and sadness" *to* "binge eating, overeating and dysregulated eating", and from "interiorized weight stigma" *to* "binge eating, overeating and dysregulated eating" and sedentary lifestyle.")

Figure 6.1 shows the patient's personal formulation constructed as described above.

After creating the personal formulation, the therapist should discuss with the patient its implications. The main point to emphasize is that in order to overcome the eating problem, and eliminate the things that the patient would like to change (e.g., binge-eating episodes, overeating, and dysregulated eating), it will be necessary to disrupt the processes that are reinforcing, or maintaining, them (the vicious

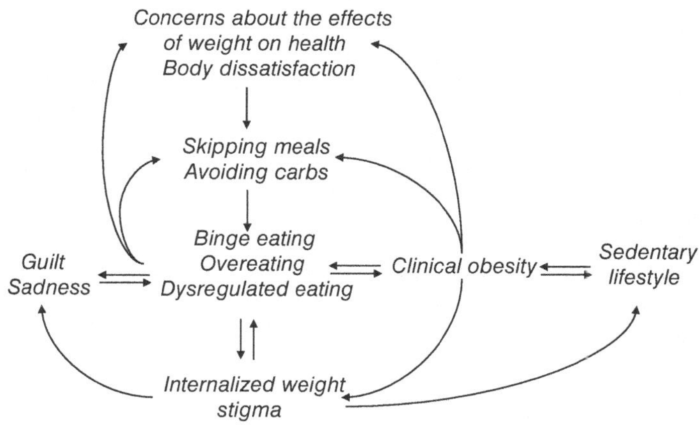

Fig. 6.1 The personal formulation of the patient with BED and clinical obesity described in the text

cycles). For example, the patient described above will need to address their extreme and rigid dieting (when trying to lose weight), concerns about weight, body dissatisfaction, internalized weight stigma, sedentary lifestyle, and events and associated mood changes, which all affect their eating. Trying to stop binge-eating episodes without eroding the maintenance mechanisms propping them up greatly increases the likelihood of relapse. The therapist might say something like this: "*This formulation is a diagram showing the main mechanisms that are maintaining your binge-eating episodes, overeating, dysregulated eating, and clinical obesity. In order for you to overcome your eating problem, we have to address all of them.*' The therapist should then introduce the goals and treatment plan, referring to the personal formulation and saying something like: '*I suggest we start by focusing on your eating habits, and then move on to address the other aspects. We should deal with one issue at a time and address your concerns about weight gain, body dissatisfaction, clinical obesity, internalized weight stigma, and events and mood influencing eating later on.*"

6.4 Informing Patients about the Treatment

Creating the personal formulation also serves as a visual prop for re-explaining the nature of CBT for BED. Although this information will have already been provided to the patient during Assessment and Preparation, in our clinical experience, it is worth repeating. Go over the items in Chap. 4 and Table 4.1 again to ensure that the patient has fully understood. It is worth focusing in particular on the following points:

- How the treatment is organized
- How many sessions are there and how long are they

- How will the be sessions conducted
- The importance of being punctual and attending all sessions
- Does the treatment focus on the processes maintaining the eating problem
- The need to play an active role in the treatment
- The need to make the treatment a priority
- That what is done between sessions is the key to recovery (homework is non-negotiable)
- The patient, not the therapist, is in charge of the treatment
- After this "orientation", the therapist should encourage the patient to ask any questions and express any concerns they may have. It is vital that the therapist ensures that the patient is fully "on board".

6.5 Introducing Real-Time Self-Monitoring

6.5.1 Rationale

Self-monitoring is a key procedure of CBT for BED. It consists of the patient self-reporting, on a dedicated monitoring record, any relevant behaviours, thoughts, emotions, and events that they may be experiencing "in the moment". Real-time self-monitoring is introduced in Session 0, after the treatment orientation. It is reviewed and refined in Session 1, and will be practised by the patient without interruption until the first part of Step Three.

Self-monitoring has two main goals [3]: (i) to help the patient and therapist improve their understanding of the eating problem according to the psychological explanation of CBT for BED, and (ii) to help the patient see that it is possible to change.

The best understanding of the eating problem comes through real-time self-monitoring. Recording relevant behaviours, thoughts, emotions, and events as they occur minimizes the memory issues that typically plague the strategy of filling in a traditional food diary at the end of meals or in the evening. In addition, it gives the patient and therapist "team" repeated opportunities to identify emerging maintenance mechanisms or barriers, and therefore to update, amend, or affirm the initial personal formulation. Self-monitoring also helps a patient to enact change, because real-time recording makes the patient more aware of what they are doing at the precise moment in which they are doing it. This facilitates the modification of behaviours that seem automatic, such as binge eating.

It is our experience that the patient's adherence to self-monitoring depends on how seriously the therapist takes this procedure. We tell the patient that it makes no sense to continue the treatment without regular self-monitoring.

6.5.2 Procedure

Real-time self-monitoring can be introduced and explained by saying something like this [4]:

"Self-monitoring is critical for your treatment. It's just as important as attending our sessions. It is the tool that will allow you and I to become experts on your eating problem and how to overcome it. Self-monitoring has two main purposes:

1. *It will allow you to accurately identify what is happening minute by minute and day by day. You and I need to know the details of what you are doing and experiencing in order to understand how we can address your eating problem. Your monitoring record can be compared to an X-ray that a dentist takes to identify the cause of your tooth pain and how best to treat it. In the same way, your monitoring record will help us better understand the mechanisms that are maintaining your eating problem, and to decide which procedures to use to interrupt them.*
2. *It will help you make beneficial changes. By becoming aware of what you are doing, thinking and feeling at the very moment when things are happening, you will learn that you have choices, and that some things that you thought were automatic and beyond your control (and perhaps you weren't aware of) can be changed with attention, effort and practice. But this can only be done if you accurately self-monitor in real time. Simply remembering how things were a few hours ago doesn't work. Real-time monitoring can be equated to looking in the mirror when learning a dance. Only if you watch what you are doing can you correct any mistakes that you would otherwise fail to notice. However, I must warn you that self-monitoring can have a negative effect in the short term. It may make you more concerned about your eating, but this effect is short-lived, and it is important to stick with it. Only then you will realize how much benefit you can get from using this procedure."*

Real-time recording is crucial for the reasons described above. However, it is challenging for some patients and requires a lot of effort. Hence, the CBT for BED monitoring record is as simple to complete and use as possible. A blank form can be found in Appendix 1, together with instructions on how to fill it in. What is recorded will evolve during treatment, and additional columns may be added as needed for some patients. Initially, however, the emphasis is mainly on the patient's eating habits and physical activity.

To facilitate their understanding of how to use the monitoring record, we point out the following aspects to the patients (described in detail in the instructions in Appendix 1):

- The various columns and what they are used to record
- How to write down the food and drinks: the patient is asked to provide a simple and non-detailed description of the amount of food and drinks they consume. They should be explicitly instructed not to weigh food or report the calorie content of what they are eating.
- How to use asterisks (to indicate each food eaten with a feeling of losing control), parentheses/brackets (to delimit main meals—not snacks or other food intake episodes).

- How to use the Comments column. At this stage of the treatment, this column is usually reserved for recording events, thoughts, and emotions that have affected eating, as well as those that are considered important, even if they were not related to eating. In addition, each time the patient weighs themself, they must write the reading on the scales in this column.
- How to count the number of steps (estimated with a pedometer or digital wristband, which the therapist will preferably provide), and the type and minutes of formal exercise (i.e., physical activity that involves exertion and increases heart and respiratory rate, such as swimming, tennis, running).

The patient should not have to worry about making spelling mistakes. It should be made clear that what is important is that the monitoring record is filled in as events occur and brought to the session, not that they are neat and well-written.

Self-monitoring in social situations (e.g., in the cafeteria at work, at a friend or relative's house, or in a restaurant) should also be discussed. It is suggested that on such occasions self-monitoring be performed using a spare piece of paper or smartphone, to be transcribed on the monitoring record when they get home or have an opportunity to distance themselves from the social situation and fill it in a secluded place, for example, when going to the bathroom. As yet we have not encountered any situation in which real-time recording was not possible.

It may be enlightening for the therapist to try self-monitoring on their own for a week to understand the difficulties encountered, and share any strategies they devise for overcoming them with their patient. It is also vital to discuss with the patient that there may be a temptation not to record binge-eating episodes out of shame and embarrassment. The point to emphasize is that, for the treatment to succeed, the patient and therapist must be aware of the problem in its entirety, so honesty is always the policy. This is an ideal opportunity to reassure the patient that they will never be judged for their eating behaviour.

It is always advisable to ask the patient if they have any questions or concerns about the prospect of starting real-time monitoring. Below are the most common queries and doubts in our experience, and suggestions on how to respond.

Patient: I've done self-monitoring before, and it didn't help at all!

Therapist: Did you use something identical to the monitoring record we discussed?

Patient: No, it was a food diary. There were no asterisks.

Therapist: Did you record in your diary the events, thoughts and emotions that influenced your eating?

Patient: No, I just made a few general comments.

Therapist: Were you advised to do monitoring in real time?

Patient: No, I kept a record of what I had eaten at the end of the meal.

Therapist: As you can see, the monitoring record that we will use is very different from the food diary you used previously because recording in real time will improve our understanding of the eating problem and help you interrupt certain behaviours, even those—like binge-eating episodes—which might seem automatic and beyond your control. Try using it over the next few days to see if it will be helpful to you.

Patient: Okay, I'll try.

Patient: It's going to increase my concerns about eating!

Therapist: True, writing down what you eat may increase your concerns about eating in the short term. However, these are constructive concerns because they help you become more aware of your problematic eating behaviour and the processes that are maintaining it. It is a necessary step if you are to fully understand on the psychological mechanisms that are making it difficult for you to overcome your eating problem. If you keep at it, you will see that your concerns about eating will taper off after a couple of weeks.

Patient: I'd be too ashamed to report what I eat and feel.

Therapist: I assure you that I will never judge your behaviours or feelings. My job is to help you find effective strategies to cope with them. For this reason, you should try to be honest and open in reporting what you do and feel on your monitoring record.

Patient: Should I use the monitoring record while eating meals?

Therapist: Yes, as I said it is important for you to record what you are eating and how you are feeling when you are doing it. You will realize that by doing so, you will be able to distance yourself from your thoughts and emotions and stop certain behaviours that seem automatic (e.g., eating too fast or too much).

Patient: Do I always need to carry the monitoring records with me?

Therapist: Yes, I recommend that you do this, even though it may sometimes be challenging. You can put your monitoring record in your pocket or wallet. It doesn't matter if it gets creased or wrinkled. It is a tool: if it is not in pristine condition, it will mean that it has been used.

Patient: How do I do real-time recording when I'm out with friends or in the cafeteria at work?

Therapist: In these situations, you can walk away from the table with the excuse that you have to make a phone call or go to the bathroom, and then write down what you have had to eat and drink and how you feel. It only takes a few moments. Or do you have a better suggestion?

Patient: Can I allow my family members to see my monitoring records?

Therapist: I advise you not to show anybody but me, because it might influence what you write. You should consider your monitoring record a confidential document for our eyes only.

At the end of this discussion, the therapist should give the patient 20 blank monitoring records with written instructions for completing them (see Appendix 1), and an example of a completed self-monitoring (Fig. 6.2). It is advisable to review each point of the instructions to make sure it is clear to the patient what they have to record and how. We generally advise patients to begin self-monitoring either immediately or the following morning. We reiterate to the patient that they should keep their monitoring records private but take them with them wherever they go so that they can update them in real time, whatever the occasion. We advise patients to file their monitoring records sequentially in a large ring binder. This will facilitate reviewing previous entries and comparing changes in eating habits and exercise over the course of treatment.

Day *13th February* **Date** *Thursday*

Time	Food and drink consumed	Place	*	Comments
7:00	*1 cappuccino* *1 sachet of sugar* *1 cream croissant*]	*Bar*		*It's my usual breakfast*
10:00	*1 coffee*	*Work*		
11:00	*1 slice of cheesecake* *1 glass of coke*	*Work*	* *	*It is Roberta's birthday, and I couldn't say no. I feel guilty. I will eat less at lunch.*
13:00	*1 tuna and mozzarella salad* *1 bottle of still water*]	*Bar*		*I was good: I didn't have any bread or dessert.*
14:30	*1 coffee* *2 packaged snacks*	*Food vending machine at work*	*	*I just wanted to get a coffee, but then I saw the snacks at the vending machine, and as usual couldn't resist.*
18:00	*1 tub of ice cream (500 g)* *10 cookies* *2 cans of orange soda*	*Kitchen*	* * *	*I felt down and frustrated and to ld myself that the day was over now and that I would stick to the diet tomorrow. I have no control over my diet*
20:00	*1 large plate of pasta with tomato* *2 slices of bread* *1 fruit*] *2 pieces of cheese* *About 20 nuts*	*Kitchen*	* *	*I ate with my husband. Then we stayed at the table chatting, and I ate the cheese and nuts without realizing it.*
22:00	*5 chocolates* *10 cookies*	*On the sofa in the living room*	* *	*When I watch TV, I always want to eat something sweet (it's a habit)*
Steps		Number: *3,250*		
Formal exercise		Type:		Minutes:

Fig. 6.2 Example of a completed monitoring record

6.6 Setting Homework for the Next Session

"Homework" is an integral part of CBT for BED and is critical to achieving change. Generally, the following homework is agreed at the end of Session 0:

1. Reviewing the personal formulation, considering what seems most relevant, what may need to be added, and what should be deleted.
2. Beginning real-time self-monitoring and carefully reading the instructions for doing so.

It is good practice to ensure that the patient writes down precisely the homework agreed upon on the back of their monitoring record. In addition, the therapist will explain the collaborative weighting procedure (see Chap. 7) to the patient and notify them that it will begin in the next session.

6.7 Summarizing the Session and Arranging the Next Appointment

As with all subsequent sessions, the therapist should end Session 0 by summarizing the session, re-stating the homework assignments, and scheduling the next appointment.

References

1. Cooper Z, Calugi S, Dalle GR. Controlling binge eating and weight: a treatment for binge eating disorder worth researching? Eat Weight Disord. 2019;25(4):1105–9. https://doi.org/10.1007/s40519-019-00734-4.
2. Dalle Grave R, Calugi S. Cognitive behavior therapy for adolescents with eating disorders. New York: Guilford Press; 2020.
3. Fairburn CG. Cognitive behavior therapy and eating disorders. New York: Guilford Press; 2008.
4. Dalle Grave R, Calugi S. A young person's guide to cognitive behaviour therapy for eating disorders. London: Routledge; 2024.

Session 1 7

Abstract

The main priority of Session 1 of cognitive behaviour therapy (CBT) for binge-eating disorder (BED) is continuing to bolster patient engagement. The session starts by initiating collaborative weighing and providing personalized information about weight and weighing, including weight regulation and interpretation. The second major goal of Session 1 is to assess and reinforce real-time self-monitoring by focusing mainly on the *process* (i.e., how the patient feels about monitoring and using the procedure) rather than on its *content*, which will be analyzed in detail over subsequent sessions. Afterwards, the Eating Problem Checklist (EPCL) for BED is introduced. This 15-item self-report measurement tool is designed to assess eating-disorder behaviours and psychopathology in patients with BED. From this point on, it should be completed once a week after a joint review of the monitoring records. Then, the session will focus on addressing low physical activity levels. The last part of the session will be dedicated to assessing the patient's attitudes towards treatment, and reviewing the personal formulation.

7.1 Structure and Content

The priority of Session 1, like that of Session 0, is patient engagement. Without their engagement, this treatment will not work. Hence, the therapist should do their best to cultivate the patient's enthusiasm, hope, and drive for change, and at the same time address, if necessary, any concerns, fears, or pessimism regarding their chances of overcoming their eating problem. The other goals of Session 1 are:

- Initiating collaborative weighing and providing personalized information about weight and weighing
- Reviewing in detail and reinforcing self-monitoring

R. Dalle Grave et al., *Cognitive Behavior Therapy for Binge Eating Disorder*, https://doi.org/10.1007/978-3-031-71456-6_7

- Introducing the Eating Problem Checklist (EPCL for BED)
- Developing an active lifestyle
- Assessing attitudes toward treatment
- Reviewing the formulation

This session, like those that follow, should last about 50 minutes and focus on examining the *process* (rather the content) of self-monitoring in detail, to establish and reinforce the optimal use of this tool. The session is structured as follows (the approximate amount of time to be devoted to each topic is indicated in brackets):

- Initiating in-session weighing (5 minutes)
- Reviewing monitoring records (about 10–15 minutes)
- Introducing the EPCL for BED (5 minutes)
- Setting the agenda for the session (a few minutes)
- Working through the items in the agenda (25 minutes)
- Summarizing the session, agreeing on homework, and arranging the next appointment (5 minutes)

7.2 Collaborative Weighing

7.2.1 Rationale

Many patients with BED have misconceptions about body weight, particularly regarding the causes of weight changes. In addition, most are concerned and dissatisfied with their weight and are anxious about the effects that treatment will have on it. This concern is reflected in how they weigh themselves, which can range from not doing it at all (weight avoidance) to weighing themselves frequently, even several times a day. Both behaviours are an obstacle to changing eating habits because they promote weight gain and, indirectly, eating concerns.

Collaborative in-session weighting is a fundamental treatment procedure designed to correct misconceptions and reduce patient concerns about weight. The procedure consists of (i) weekly weighing and recording, and (ii) personalized education about weight and weighing. The strategy has five main goals [1]:

1. To correct misconceptions about weight and weighing
2. To address either frequent weighing or weight avoidance
3. To provide patients with reliable information about their own weight
4. To help patients interpret the number on the scales correctly
5. To reduce weight and eating concerns

7.2.2 Procedure

Session 1 begins with collaborative weighing, in which the therapist and patient jointly check the patient's weight (with the latter wearing indoor clothing and no shoes). We use scales with a half-kilogram range, not medical or electronic scales with 100 g ranges, because their apparently greater accuracy fuels patients' concerns about minor changes in weight. Collaborative weighing is performed weekly, in session, and the patient is asked to cease weighing themselves at home (if applicable). The therapist must address their concerns about this, and the collaborative weighing procedure itself.

Few adult patients with BED are reluctant to be weighed or agree only on the condition that they are not told their weight, sometimes asking that weighing be postponed until the following week, hoping that they will lose weight in the interim. There must be an agreement on collaborative weighing from Session 1 to ensure that this procedure is implemented consistently, without becoming a point of discussion during treatment. Hence, if a patient is reluctant to begin, it is essential to emphasize that regular weighing will help them feel in control and reduce their concerns about weight. What you do not know is often more frightening than what you do.

Weighing should be as collaborative as possible, with the therapist adopting a calm, non-judgemental attitude. The reading on the scales should be acknowledged and spoken aloud by the therapist, thus counteracting any possible avoidance of the patient knowing their own weight. The patient should be asked to note this number in an individualized weight chart (a graph the therapist will have prepared in advance using the blank weight chart like that in Appendix 2). From the next session onwards, at the beginning of each session, the patient will be collaboratively weighed and asked to enter the weight measured and interpret any result. Naturally, this interpretation is impossible in Session 1, as only one reading has been made. Nevertheless, this should be the session in which the patient is educated on when to measure their weight and how it should be interpreted (see below).

7.3 Providing Personalized Information about Weight and Weighing

7.3.1 Information about Weight Regulation

The first topic is to educate the patient on weight regulation. The main information to be given is the following [1–3]:

- Our body weight is strongly influenced by our genetics [4, 5], so changing it significantly in the long term is challenging. Indeed, our body weight is not regulated around a fixed point, as was initially thought, because in Western countries body weight tends to increase with age. The more recent theories (e.g., the dual intervention-point model) postulate that there is an upper and lower physiological intervention point (probably influenced by genetics) that hamper further weight gain or loss, respectively. According to the set-point theory, the human body has a predetermined range of fat mass [6]. Various compensatory physiological mechanisms maintain the upper and lower limits of that range and oppose any deviation from it. In other words, we can make lifestyle changes to alter our body weight within this range, but this is regulated by environmental pressures (see Fig. 7.1) [7]. Although this is not entirely clear, the body weight range that is not hindered by potent physiological pressure seems to be between 5% and 10%. In short, the biological odds are stacked against losing more than 5–10% of body weight.

- The number on the scales fluctuates throughout the day due to changes in the body's hydration status, which accounts for about 60% of body weight. Bowel and bladder content, the phase of the menstrual cycle, and other factors are also influence "water weight", but changes in hydration status, not fat, are the main cause of short-term weight fluctuations.
- Physiological fluctuations in weight make it almost impossible to keep body weight at a fixed point. Generally, to allow for natural weight fluctuations it is advisable to accept a weight range of about 3 kg (rather than a fixed point) without changing the energy intake.

To help patients understand and accept normal fluctuations in weight, the therapist might say something like this:

Therapist: Wanting to be the same weight all the time is like wanting the same heart rate or body temperature all the time. Do you think it is possible?

Patient: No, it's impossible.

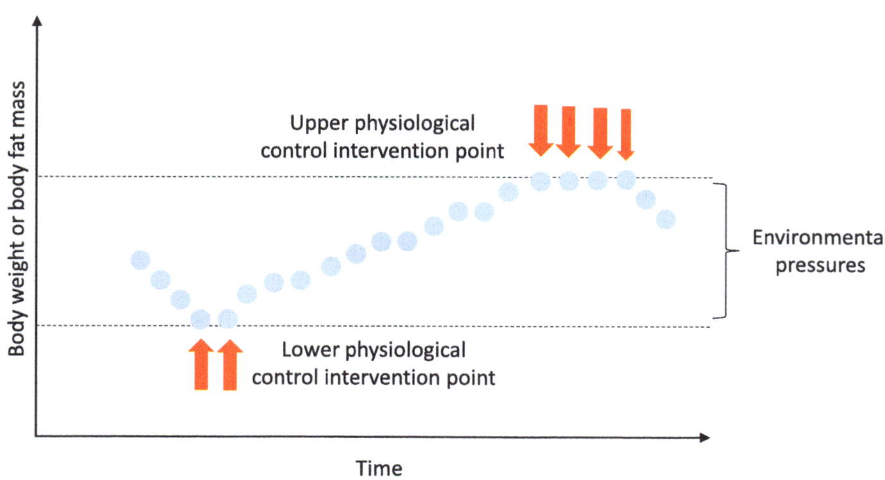

Fig. 7.1 A schematic model of the dual intervention point model on body weight and body fat regulation

Therapist: That's right. Our heartbeat changes when our circumstances change, like when we exercise or experience intense emotions. This is not something we can alter. Similarly, our weight is affected by changes in our body's water content, which makes up about 60% of our weight.

Patient: Okay.

7.3.2 Information about Weight Interpretation

The second topic is to educate the patient on how to interpret weight changes. The main information to be given are the following [1]:

- People tend to misinterpret fluctuations in weight as changes in body fat, when they are mainly due to variations in their hydration status.
- Focusing on a single reading can be misleading and not necessarily related to stable changes in body weight.
- To correctly interpret weight changes, it is necessary to look at the trend over 4 weeks. If the current weight and those from the previous 3 weeks on the weight graph are connected using a transparent ruler, what do they show? Is the weight fluctuating or tending to increase or decrease?

Going by this rule, weight change can only be interpreted correctly from the fourth session onwards. Still, at this stage the therapist should use collaborative weighing to reinforce the procedure remind the patient that it is impossible to interpret a single reading on the scales. It may also be helpful to practice weight interpretation in session, as reported in the following transcript (see also Fig. 7.2).

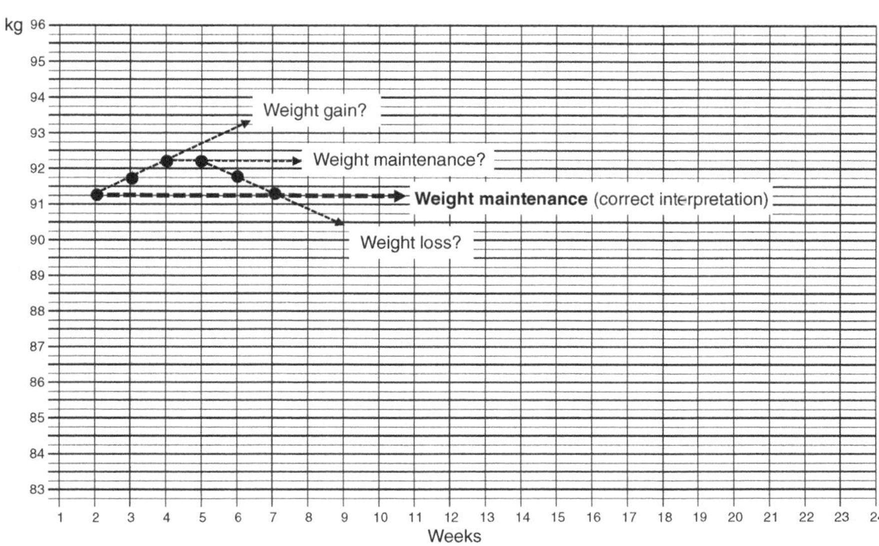

Fig 7.2 Example of the weight interpretation exercise described in the text

Therapist: Do you mind if we do an exercise to practice interpreting weight changes in a person of your age, whom we will call Anna?

Patient: Okay.

Therapist: Anna weighed herself four weeks ago, and the number on the scales was 90 kg. Can you put a black circle on 90 kg in week 1 of this weight chart?

Patient: Okay.

Therapist: The following week, Anna weighed herself again and got a reading of 90.5 kg. Can you mark it in week 2?

Patient: Okay.

Therapist: Then, in weeks 3 and 4, the scale said 91 kg, while it said 90.5 kg in week 5 and 90 kg in week 6. Can you please mark these on the weight graph?

Patient: Of course, it's not difficult.

Therapist: What would you conclude if you were to evaluate Anna's weight trend after the measurements in weeks 2 and 3?

Patient: That she has put on 1 kg.

Therapist: Okay. And how would you assess the trend between weeks 3 and 4?

Patient: Her weight remained stable.

Therapist: What about between weeks 4 and 6?

Patient: She lost weight.

Therapist: Please assess the weight trend from week 1 to week 6. Use this ruler and draw a dotted line. What do you conclude?

Patient: Anna's weight remained stable.

Therapist: Yes, that's right. As you can see from the graph, none of the individual interpretations were correct because they only referred to the change in weight from one week to the next. To understand if your body weight is going up or down, or fluctuating but stable as in Anna's case, it is not possible to interpret a single reading. You need to assess the weight trend over the last four to five weeks.

Patient: Yes, that is clear.

7.3.3 Information About Weighing

The third and final component of collaborative weighing is to educate the patient about weight checking and avoidance. Many patients with BED and clinical obesity (see Sect. 4.3.1 and Table 4.4 for the definition) tend to avoid weighing themselves or, especially during periods of weight loss, check their weight frequently. Both behaviours contribute to maintaining excessive concerns about weight. Avoiding weighing does not provide any information about weight changes, allowing weight to increase or decrease without control. Like an ostrich burying its head in the sand, there is no way to escape from impending danger, but also no way to reassure oneself that one is safe. In addition to not mitigating fears and assumptions about weight, avoidance facilitates the maintenance of overeating and dysregulated eating. At the other end of the spectrum, weighing oneself frequently—every day or several times a day—stimulates concerns about insignificant changes secondary to changes in "water weight", and encourages dysfunctional dieting. Alternatively, it may prompt the reaction of temporary abandonment of eating control associated with all-or-nothing thinking (e.g., "*My efforts have been for nothing because I have gained weight; I might as well give up and eat what I want*".).

The therapist can use the above example of heart rate measurement to help patients understand the futility and potential negative consequences of not weighing themselves or weighing themselves frequently. A sample script for this is provided below:

Therapist: Try to imagine what would happen to a person who is concerned about their heart if they measured their heart rate several times a day. What effect might frequent heart rate checking have?

Patient: I don't know… Maybe they would get worried when their heart rate goes up.

Therapist: Yes, you're right. They would get worried, and might even think they are about to have a heart attack. This effect happens because repeated checking of heart rate can lead to interpreting natural changes in heart rate as something abnormal in heart functioning. In other words, repeated measurement of the heart rate in this person could accentuate and maintain their concerns of having a diseased heart.

Patient: Yes, that sounds right.

Therapist: On the other hand, never measuring our heart rate would not enable us to tell if our heart were beating too fast or abnormally, which would be equally unhelpful.

Patient: Yes, checking your pulse occasionally can be helpful.

Therapist: If you think about it, the same applies to checking weight. If it is too frequent, it leads to greater concerns about changes in weight, when it is in actual fact only fluctuating due to hydration status. Weight cannot be interpreted on the basis of a single reading. In the same way, never weighing oneself does not provide reliable information on weight changes, and therefore the belief that weight is increasing cannot be disproved. This only leads to more fear of weighing.

Patient: Yes, that's right.

A central aspect of collaborative weighing, and the treatment itself, is to help the patient learn how to weigh themselves with a frequency that allows them to accurately understand if their weight has changed, without increasing their concerns about weight and eating. According to our clinical experience, once-a-week weighing strikes the right balance, and for this reason, we ask patients to resist the urge to weigh themselves at home and to collaboratively measure and interpret their weight once a week.

If a patient finds it challenging to resist the urge to weigh themselves between sessions, it is advisable for them to make a "coping card" on which they write why it is not worth, for the moment, weighing themselves at home. If they are unable to resist the urge to weigh themselves, they should report their weight in the Comments column on their monitoring record, along with the events, thoughts, and emotions that led them to check their weight.

In our experience, weekly collaborative weighing and interpretation have the effect of reducing weight concerns, and consequently disrupting a key mechanism that maintains dysfunctional dietary restriction, overeating, dysregulating eating, and binge-eating episodes. As a guide to implementing this procedure, below is a transcript in which the therapist addresses weight avoidance by a patient.

Therapist: As we said in the previous session, we will start collaborative weighing today. How do you feel about that?

Patient: Terrible. I don't want to weigh myself.

Therapist: I understand. What worries you about weighing yourself now?

Patient: I don't want to see how I've ended up.

Therapist: When you say, "how I've ended up", are you referring to your weight?

Patient: Yes. If I see how much I weigh, I will get even more depressed, and I already know that I have let myself go.

Therapist: I understand what you mean, and acknowledge your fear of knowing how much you weigh. However, I would like to discuss the risks of avoiding knowing your weight. Let's try to take the perspective of beginning treatment without knowing anything about the starting point. How are we going to figure out how things are going?

Patient: We can see if I am eating properly from the monitoring record and how I feel about my body when I wear clothes. I know if I'm controlling my weight by how my clothes fit!

Therapist: I get it. However, let's consider this situation: how would you react if you had a day when you ate more than you planned?

Patient: I would be worried.

Therapist: What would you be worried about?

Patient: Well, I would have eaten too much and therefore not lost any weight!

Therapist: So, how would you cope with that concern?

Patient: In my experience, I would react by trying to skip meals and avoid carbs for a few days… or get so discouraged that I would binge and think I would never be able to lose weight!

Therapist: So, if I have understood correctly, either you would follow a strict diet or binge. Can you confirm this?

Patient: Yes!

Therapist: So, in the second case, the reaction would be the same as the one you gave about the idea of starting collaborative weighing: getting depressed because of how you've ended up?

Patient: Yes, that's right!

Therapist: So, it wouldn't change anything!

Patient: Indeed!

Therapist: Yes, because your eating concerns (*the therapist indicates* "eating concerns" *on the patient's formulation*) make you interpret even the slightest change in diet as a total loss of control, leading you to abandon all attempts to maintain a flexible, healthy eating pattern. However, weekly collaborative weighing can alleviate your concerns about eating, because knowing your weight and how it is actually changing will help you to understand that weight cannot be affected by tiny dietary changes. This procedure will help you reduce your concerns about eating and, as a result, develop better control of your eating and weight.

Patient: Yes, but I'll know I have gained weight, even if I haven't weighed myself.

Therapist: It might be true. You told me that you might react to putting on weight by severely restricting your diet. In your opinion, are there any potential risks to that reaction?

Patient: Uhm... yes, I it is hard and tiring to always to follow a strict diet because I must always be careful not to lose control.

Therapist: Any other risks?

Patient: I don't think so.

Therapist: From what you have told me, and as we have seen from your formulation, extreme and rigid food restriction makes binge-eating episodes more likely, it maintains them.

Patient: Oh yes, of course!

Therapist: So, again, if you act on your concerns and restrict your diet, this will only increase the risk you will have a binge-eating episode. We will talk about your beliefs about certain foods in a later session, but for the moment, do you think that this all-or-nothing attitude towards eating control is helpful?

Patient: Not if you put it like that, no.

Therapist: As for using how your body feels to understand how much you weigh, I would say that that is also a risky strategy because these sensations are influenced by many situations, for example feeling full, which is normal after having eaten, or changing position, which may make your clothes feel tight. These are not reliable signals that your weight is changing over time.

Patient: I understand...

Therapist: At this point, I think you have two alternatives: either continue not to weigh yourself, with the risk of continuing to have binge-eating episodes and gaining weight, or start weekly collaborative weighing with me and learning to interpret your weight and any changes, which is an important part of your treatment.

Patient: I guess. I don't seem to have any choice!

Therapist: Naturally, the first time we do this you might feel anxious, but I assure you that it will get easier over time if we continue to measure and interpret your weight together in the weekly sessions. I am convinced that starting collaborative weighing today is the lesser of two evils.

Patient: Okay, I'll give it a go.

Therapist: You'll see that you won't regret it. Can we proceed then?

Patient: Yes, okay.

7.4 Reviewing and Reinforcing Monitoring

The second main goal of Session 1 is to assess how real-time monitoring is going and reinforce the procedure. At this point, the main focus should be on the process, how the procedure is done, rather than on the content, which will be analyzed in detail in subsequent sessions. The patient should be invited to explain to the therapist how they filled in their monitoring records since Session 0 (usually there will be three or four monitoring records to review), a process that, if done well, will take 10–15 minutes. To assess the quality of self-monitoring, the therapist must pay attention to the following aspects [1]:

- How the patient feels about it
- How they think it has been going
- Whether they had any problems with it
- How long after eating and/or drinking they recorded the relevant information
- Whether they neglected to record anything
- Whether brackets and asterisks have been used correctly

The patient must be praised for their efforts even if the monitoring records have some flaws. For example, the therapist might say, "*This is a great start. I can imagine how challenging it was to fill out the monitoring records. What we need to do now is to talk about what you can improve to get the most out of them. What do you think about this suggestion…?*"

If a patient comes to Session 1 without having recorded anything since the last session, the best thing to do is to explore the underlying reasons with them. One strategy we generally use is to take responsibility for the problem, saying something like this: "*I don't think I explained to you why it is so important for you to do self-monitoring in real time or how to do it properly. Do you mind if we go over it again?*"

Then, the therapist should address any issues that emerge from this discussion. It is important to reiterate that self-monitoring is an essential part of treatment, which has no chance of success without it. We have found that in all cases this explanation is sufficient to get patients to start monitoring. We have experienced that adherence to this procedure depends mainly on the therapist's success in conveying to the patient the utility of the practice of self-monitoring in real time. This does not however, exclude the possibility that there may be problems we have not encountered, or that issues may arise during treatment.

7.5 Introducing the EPCL for BED

After collaborative weighing, weight education, and a review of the monitoring records, the Eating Problem Check List for BED (EPCL-BED) (see Appendix 3 and Table A2) should be introduced. The therapist should explain to the patients how to use the questionnaire, a 15-item self-report measurement tool designed to assess eating-disorder behaviours and psychopathology in patients with BED, every week. It should be completed once a week after the joint review of the monitoring records. The therapist should explain to the patients that it is important that the EPCL-BED is completed truthfully and accurately, because their responses will enable the therapist and patient to jointly assess the improvements achieved and the obstacles encountered each week. Based on this assessment, the patient's personal formulation can be updated, and any dysfunctional behaviours and attitudes can be identified and addressed. The information that the questionnaire reveals should be recorded on the Weekly Changes Summary Spreadsheet (see Appendix 3 and Table A3). This will allow collaborative assessment of the changes, as described in Chap. 9 ("Reviewing the EPCL-BED").

7.6 Addressing Low Physical Activity

Exercise plays a critical role in the management of patients with BED associated with clinical obesity. Exercise is also one of the most influential behaviours on long-term weight maintenance [8], and is associated with significant reductions in the incidence of cardiovascular events both in general [9] and in high-risk groups [10]. It also has a protective effect against metabolic diseases (e.g., metabolic syndrome and type 2 diabetes), and it reduces the visceral accumulation of adipose tissue, as well as triglyceride levels, blood pressure, and the risk of mortality [11].

A patient's commitment to increasing their level of physical activity can be fostered by providing the following main reasons for doing so:

- It improves health. Specifically, it cuts the risk of cardiovascular disease and mortality, reducing cardiovascular risk factors, regardless of weight loss [12]. Numerous studies have shown that people with clinical obesity who adopt an active lifestyle have, compared to those who diet to lose weight, a greater reduced risk of cardiovascular disease and premature death [13].
- It helps a person cope with mood changes without eating or binges. Evidence suggests that physical activity can help weight control by improving the balance between food intake and energy expenditure (an action that regulates food intake—an important effect in people with BED) or by increasing energy expenditure so that it is difficult for people to achieve a positive energy balance through food intake [14]. Although physical activity without calorie reduction may cause a small weight loss (2–3 kg), it is more important for long-term weight maintenance [15].

- It improves body image and psychological well-being. In clinical trials of physical activity interventions, participants reported better body image and greater psychological well-being afterwards than participants in control groups who did not exercise [16].

7.6.1 Assessing Individual Activity Levels and Obstacles to Change

The therapist should empathetically assess how the patient judges their current level of physical activity, and whether they feel it is enough to maintain a healthy lifestyle. If, as is often the case, the patient reports being sedentary, they should be asked about the reasons for their sedentary lifestyle, and if there are any barriers to their exercising. In general, most obstacles reported by our patients include low motivation and perceived lack of self-efficacy, no history of exercise, inadequate access to gyms or other facilities, the high cost of training programmes, low social and cultural support, and time constraints [17]. Other obstacles more specific to individuals with BED and clinical obesity include low fitness, poor physical condition (e.g., arthritis, obstructive sleep apnoea), shame associated with body exposure, and fear of injury or death. If BED is also associated with clinical depression, the low mood and asthenia often associated with it are an additional major obstacle to exercise.

7.6.2 Actively Involving the Patient in the Decision to Change

The therapist should encourage patients to consider their motivations for and against exercise. To have a handy reference for the future, it is useful to have these written down. We therefore recommend that a "pros and cons of change" table (see the example in Table 7.1) be collaboratively created. It is best to start by asking the patient to list the negative aspects of making a change: whether a sedentary lifestyle offers them any perceived benefits that they would be reluctant or afraid to give up. Subsequently, the patient should be asked to write down the benefits of taking up

Table 7.1 An example of the pros and cons of change table

Reasons not to exercise	Reasons to exercise
I'll have to do it even when I don't feel like it	*I'll be better able to control my weight*
I'll have to get over my laziness	*I'll feel good psychologically*
I like to rest when I have some free time	*It will help me manage emotions without binge eating*
I get exhausted when I exercise	*I'll be able to meet new people*
I will have less time for my hobbies	*My physical health will improve*
I'll be tired the whole time	*I'll feel fitter*
I'll be ashamed if other people see me exercising	

exercise, and then to weigh up their pros and cons. At this stage, we encourage the patient to reflect on the short- and long-term effects of exercise on their physical and psychological quality of life, and their ability to control their eating and weight. Every reason for the change must be reinforced: the goal is to help the patient conclude that exercise will be necessary to control their weight in the long term and reduce the medical and psychosocial complications associated with clinical obesity.

7.6.3 Recommended Exercise to Increase Physical Activity Levels

One of the main goals of the treatment is to help the patient gradually develop an active lifestyle, focusing first on physical activities that are part of daily life (such as walking, standing, climbing stairs, cleaning the house, and gardening) since this form of exercise helps improve body composition and cardiorespiratory fitness and is associated with better maintenance of lost weight [18]. However, lifestyle activities alone do not improve other important components of fitness, such as muscle strength (i.e., the muscle's ability to exert force against resistance), endurance (the ability to perform a specific muscle action over an extended period), body composition (the percentages of fat mass and lean mass), flexibility (the ability to move joints effectively through a full range of motion), or neuromotor fitness (the ability of the nervous system to communicate with the musculoskeletal system, which affects balance, coordination, and agility) [19]. For this reason, we recommend that the patient combine an active lifestyle with simple exercises to improve specific areas of fitness.

Formal exercise is a term we use to describe any physical activity that involves physical exertion and produces an increase in heart and breathing rate (such as swimming, tennis, running). Although formal exercise is associated with improved general health conditions, we suggest it only to those patients who are motivated to start it or take it up again.

Adherence to exercise increases when its structure is less rigid. Hence, the exercise recommended as part of the treatment focuses primarily on helping patients increase the level of physical activity involved in their daily activities. It is important that the therapist work with the patient to reduce any barriers to exercise (e.g., lack of time or financial resources) that they may perceive [20].

7.6.3.1 Reducing Sedentary Behaviour

The first strategy for developing an active lifestyle that we suggest to patients is to reduce sedentary activities. There are many ways in which this can be achieved (see Table 7.2), and strategies should be tailored to the patient's lifestyle and habits. For example, a homemaker with clinical obesity might be encouraged to spend less time watching TV, taking the stairs instead of using the elevator, and cleaning the house alone, without resorting to a housekeeper. Similarly, a person who always uses the car to get around should be encouraged to drive as little as possible and start getting around on foot or by bike.

Table 7.2 Strategies for reducing sedentary activities

At home	
	Don't use a machine if you can do it by hand (e.g., mixing food, washing the car, opening cans, mowing the lawn, etc.).
	Walk up and down the stairs several times a day.
	Do some gardening.
	Clean the house.
At work	
	Take the stairs instead of the elevator.
	Take a walk during breaks.
	Lift yourself up from your chair with your hands (if sitting for many hours a day).
Transportation	
	Walk rather than take the car.
	Park as far away from your destination as possible.
	Avoid shortcuts: take the long way round.

The patient should be informed that developing an active lifestyle through reducing sedentary activities has several positive consequences. In addition, it is easy to adopt, takes little time, does not require specific clothing or equipment, quickly becomes a habit over time, and helps a person feel physically and psychologically better.

7.6.3.2 Increasing the Number of Daily Steps

As an integral part of adopting an active lifestyle, the second strategy we suggest to patients is that they gradually increase their number of daily steps until they reach the goal of 10,000–12,000 steps per day. This exercise is easy, simple to monitor, and helps maintain muscle mass and body weight [21]. Note, however, that the patient should be discouraged from increasing the number of daily steps too quickly, as this can cause skeletal muscle pain and a rapid return to a sedentary lifestyle. One action plan that may be suggested to the patient is to use a pedometer/fitness tracker to check their usual daily step count (i.e., the number of steps at baseline) and then gradually increase their daily steps each week (e.g., the first week 5000 steps per day, the second week 7500 steps per day, and the third week 10,000 or more per day).

Regarding the intensity of the walk, we tell patients that they should walk without hyperventilating, and be able to have a conversation while walking, and not feel any musculoskeletal pain.

Discussing when to walk during the day with the patient is also advisable. We suggest that any time of the day is suitable for walking (e.g., before breakfast, after lunch, during breaks, at the end of the day before going home and/or after dinner, or late at night before going to bed) and that the patient should choose a time compatible with their lifestyle. The patient should be advised to plan when to walk and how long for, and adhere to this plan without being influenced by thoughts, emotions or physical states until this behaviour becomes a habit. Walking can also be replaced by jogging (20–40 min/day), cycling or swimming (45–60 min/day), depending on the patient's preferences.

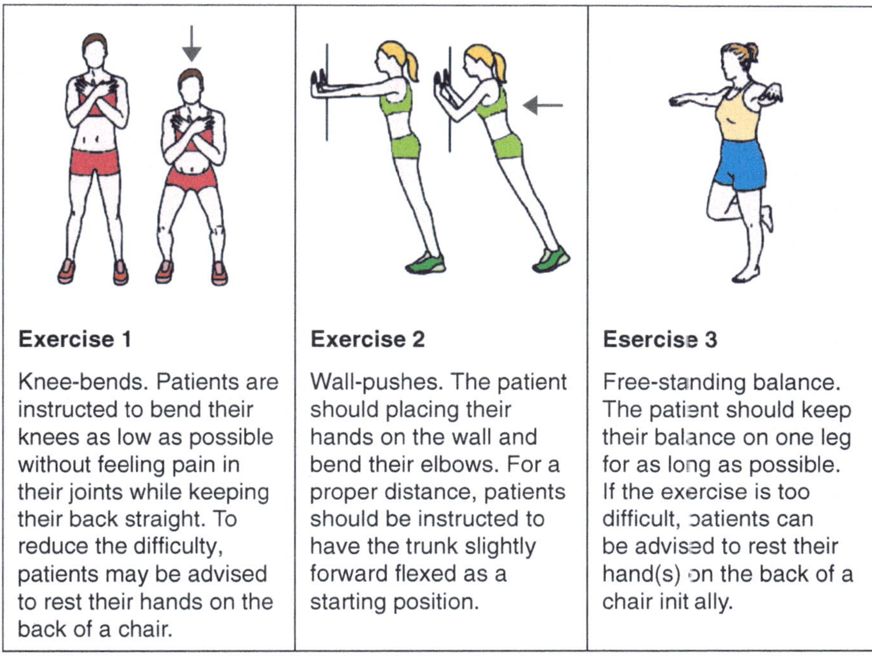
Exercise 1
Knee-bends. Patients are instructed to bend their knees as low as possible without feeling pain in their joints while keeping their back straight. To reduce the difficulty, patients may be advised to rest their hands on the back of a chair.
Exercise 2
Wall-pushes. The patient should placing their hands on the wall and bend their elbows. For a proper distance, patients should be instructed to have the trunk slightly forward flexed as a starting position.
Esercise 3
Free-standing balance. The patient should keep their balance on one leg for as long as possible. If the exercise is too difficult, patients can be advised to rest their hand(s) on the back of a chair initially.

Fig. 7.3 Three simple exercises to improve physical fitness in patients with binge-eating disorder. (Reprinted with permission (From Dalle Grave et al. [22]. Reprinted with the permission of Springer-Nature))

7.6.3.3 Improving Physical Fitness

Few clinical eating disorder teams have the opportunity to collaborate with a physical activity specialist. However, we have worked together with our team's expert on physical activity to devise three simple exercises (described in Fig. 7.3) that can be recommended to most patients with BED and clincial obesity [22]. These exercises are easy to perform and implement in everyday life, and the patient should be encouraged to perform them several times during the day. No exact number of repetitions should be set, but the patient should continue each exercise until they feel that the muscles involved are tired. However, it is always important to tell the patient not to exert themselves too early. Patients that are highly motivated to improve their cardiorespiratory, musculoskeletal, and neuromotor fitness should be assisted by a physical activity specialist who has experience working with heavier people and can suggest specific exercises.

7.6.3.4 Strategies for Continuing or Beginning Formal Exercise

Patients can gain significant health benefits by taking up formal exercise. However, most people with BED and clinical obesity have difficulty playing sports, often due to medical problems (e.g., osteoarthritis of the knees or hip) and/or feelings of embarrassment at showing their bodies to others. If a patient is willing to take up a sport or already does one, encouraging them is a good idea because exercise effectively improves overall health [23]. Nonetheless, the patient should be informed that once a sport has been undertaken, they should continue it since abrupt suspension is often associated with weight gain.

The patient who wants to take up a sport but does not have a precise idea of which to choose should be asked to write a list of sports they would like to do and evaluate the pros and cons of each, thinking about potential obstacles to be overcome (e.g., lack of time, not enough space, the need to purchase specific clothing and equipment). It is also helpful to encourage the patient to exercise with a family member or friend, join a club or gym, buy a stationary bike, etc., or take classes with a personal trainer, as these are all excellent strategies that can help the patient increase their adherence to regular sports. Note, however, that if one of our patients is reluctant to take up a sport, we do not insist, since formal exercise is not the goal of the programme.

7.7 Assessing Attitudes Toward Treatment

Patients vary in their attitude towards treatment. Some are positive from the start and remain so, whereas others start with reluctance or ambivalence but ultimately get fully involved. Some begin with enthusiasm but then lose it, while others remain reluctant or ambivalent. Changes in patient attitudes are important because they can affect the treatment outcome. Patients who start with enthusiasm tend to apply the agreed procedures with commitment, and, in most cases, see the benefits quickly. Ambivalent ones, on the other hand, often use procedures inconsistently and, as a result, make less progress and withdraw from treatment more frequently. For all these reasons, the therapist should always consider and regularly assess the patient's attitude toward treatment, asking questions like the following: "*How do you feel now that you have started treatment?*" "*Do you have any concerns or doubts about the treatment that you want to discuss?*"

7.8 Reviewing the Formulation and Continuing Education on Maintenance Mechanisms

The therapist should ask the patient if they have thought about their personal formulation and, if so, whether they think that any changes should be made. It is helpful to ascertain whether the patient has understood the meaning of the arrows (the maintenance mechanisms), particularly how dysfunctional dietary restriction and events and associated mood changes tend to maintain binge-eating episodes, and to ask whether they have any questions. This allows the personal formulation to be revised and the patient to be educated on their eating problem and the mechanisms that need to be addressed during the treatment.

7.9 Summarizing the Session, Setting the Homework, and Arranging the Next Appointment

At the end of Session 1, three homework tasks are typically agreed upon: (i) taking specific steps to improve monitoring, (ii) resisting at-home weighing, and (iii) increasing physical activity levels. The therapist should end the session by summarizing the content, going over the homework, and arranging the next appointment (see transcript below).

Therapist: May we review what we covered this session?

Patient: Yes, that's fine.

Therapist: Thank you. We started with collaborative weighing, then talked about physiological weight regulation, how to interpret weight, and the adverse effects of frequent weighing and weight avoidance.

Patient: Yes, that was interesting information, although I'm worried about my high weight.

Therapist: We reviewed your monitoring records thoroughly and concluded that you did a good job. Your records provided a lot of helpful information.

Patient: Thank you.

Therapist: You told me it was hard initially, but you're getting used to it. Is that right?

Patient: Yes.

Therapist: Then, we discussed the benefits of exercise and how to increase your physical activity levels.

Patient: Yes. I know that it is important.

Therapist: What else did we do in this session… You told me you were happy to have started the treatment and found the personalized formulation helpful.

Patient: Yes, that's true, mainly because it explains the mechanisms that maintain my binge eating.

Therapist: Good. And the last thing we decided was that you would continue to self-monitor in real time, count your daily steps, take the stairs instead of the elevator, take a walk during your morning and afternoon breaks at work, and try not to weigh yourself at home, as we will check your weekly weight together next session.

Patient: Yes, that's right.

Therapist: Okay. If you agree, I'll see you on Tuesday at three o'clock.

Patient: Okay.

References

1. Fairburn CG. Cognitive behavior therapy and eating disorders. New York: Guilford Press; 2008.
2. Dalle Grave R, Sartirana M, El Ghoch M, Calugi S. Treating obesity with personalized cognitive behavioral therapy. Cham: Springer; 2018.

3. Dalle Grave R, Calugi S. A young person's guide to cognitive behaviour therapy for eating disorders. London: Routledge; 2024.
4. Loos RJF, Yeo GSH. The genetics of obesity: from discovery to biology. Nat Rev Genet. 2022;23(2):120–33. https://doi.org/10.1038/s41576-021-00414-z.
5. Mahmoud R, Kimonis V, Butler MG. Genetics of obesity in humans: a clinical review. Int J Mol Sci. 2022;23(19) https://doi.org/10.3390/ijms231911005.
6. Kennedy GC. The role of depot fat in the hypothalamic control of food intake in the rat. Proc R Soc Lond B Biol Sci. 1953;140(901):578–96. https://doi.org/10.1098/rspb.1953.0009.
7. Speakman JR, Levitsky DA, Allison DB, Bray MS, de Castro JM, Clegg DJ, et al. Set points, settling points and some alternative models: theoretical options to understand how genes and environments combine to regulate body adiposity. Dis Model Mech. 2011;4(6):733–45.
8. Wing RR, Phelan S. Long-term weight loss maintenance. Am J Clin Nutr. 2005;82(1 Suppl):222S–5S. https://doi.org/10.1093/ajcn/82.1.222S.
9. Manson JE, Greenland P, LaCroix AZ, Stefanick ML, Mouton CP, Oberman A, et al. Walking compared with vigorous exercise for the prevention of cardiovascular events in women. N Eng J Med. 2002;347(10):716–25. https://doi.org/10.1056/NEJMoa021067.
10. Richardson CR, Kriska AM, Lantz PM, Hayward RA. Physical activity and mortality across cardiovascular disease risk groups. Med Sci Sports Exerc. 2004;36(11):1923–9. https://doi.org/10.1249/01.mss.0000145443.02568.7a.
11. Katzmarzyk PT, Church TS, Janssen I, Ross R, Blair SN. Metabolic syndrome, obesity, and mortality: impact of cardiorespiratory fitness. Diabetes Care. 2005;28(2):391–7. https://doi.org/10.2337/diacare.28.2.391.
12. Howden EJ, Leano R, Petchey W, Coombes JS, Isbel NM, Marwick TH. Effects of exercise and lifestyle intervention on cardiovascular function in CKD. Clin J Am Soc Nephrol. 2013;8(9):1494–501. https://doi.org/10.2215/cjn.10141012.
13. Barry VW, Baruth M, Beets MW, Durstine JL, Liu J, Blair SN. Fitness vs. fatness on all-cause mortality: a meta-analysis. Prog Cardiovasc Dis. 2014;56(4):382–90. https://doi.org/10.1016/j.pcad.2013.09.002.
14. Blundell JE, King NA. Physical activity and regulation of food intake: current evidence. Med Sci Sports Exerc. 1999;31(11 Suppl):S573–S83. https://doi.org/10.1097/00005768-199911001-00015.
15. Elmaleh-Sachs A, Schwartz JL, Bramante CT, Nicklas JM, Gudzune KA, Jay M. Obesity management in adults: a review. JAMA. 2023;330(20):2000–15. https://doi.org/10.1001/jama.2023.19897.
16. Andersen RE, Wadden TA, Bartlett SJ, Zemel B, Verde TJ, Franckowiak SC. Effects of lifestyle activity vs structured aerobic exercise in obese women: a randomized trial. JAMA. 1999;281(4):335–40. https://doi.org/10.1001/jama.281.4.335.
17. Sherwood NE, Jeffery RW. The behavioral determinants of exercise: implications for physical activity interventions. Annu Rev Nutr. 2000;20:21–44. https://doi.org/10.1146/annurev.nutr.20.1.21.
18. Jakicic JM, Rogers RJ. Exercise in the management of obesity. In: Brownell KD, Walsh BT, editors. Eating disorders and obesity: a comprehensive handbook. 3rd ed. New York: Guilford Press; 2017. p. 546–50.
19. Caspersen CJ, Powell KE, Christenson GM. Physical activity, exercise, and physical fitness: definitions and distinctions for health-related research. Public Health Rep (Washington, DC : 1974). 1985;100(2):126–31.
20. Fabricatore AN. Behavior therapy and cognitive-behavioral therapy of obesity: is there a difference? J Am Diet Assoc. 2007;107(1):92–9. https://doi.org/10.1016/j.jada.2006.10.005.
21. Dalle Grave R, Calugi S, El Ghoch M. Increasing adherence to diet and exercise through cognitive behavioural strategies. In: Lenzi A, Migliaccio S, Donini LM, editors. Multidisciplinary approach to obesity. Springer International Publishing; 2015. p. 327–335.

22. Dalle Grave R, Sartirana M, El Ghoch M, Calugi S. Module 4: addressing obstacles to weight loss. Treating obesity with personalized cognitive behavioral therapy. Cham: Springer; 2018. p. 89–115.
23. Warburton DE, Nicol CW, Bredin SS. Health benefits of physical activity: the evidence. CMAJ. 2006;174(6):801–9. https://doi.org/10.1503/cmaj.051351.

Session 2

8

Abstract

Session 2 of cognitive behaviour therapy (CBT) for binge-eating disorder (BED) is mainly dedicated to reviewing and reinforcing real-time monitoring, and introducing regular eating. From Session 2 onwards, the former primarily focuses on the *content* of monitoring, which helps both the patient and therapist increase their understanding of the maintenance processes acting in the patient's eating disorder, and amend or update their personalized formulation. Regular eating is concerned with the patient's eating patterns, i.e., *when* they eat rather than what or how much, and has two components: (i) eating at regular intervals throughout the day, i.e., three planned meals and two snacks, and (ii) not eating between planned meals and snacks. The procedure, if well done, rapidly reduces the frequency of binge-eating episodes and, thanks to it, at the end of Step One, most patients report only "residual" binge-eating episodes to be addressed during Step Two. To facilitate the implementation of regular eating, the patient should be advised to plan three meals and two snacks, and self-monitor eating in real time, and taught how to use the "things to say and do" procedure to cope with the urge to deviate from the eating plan, reduce food stimuli, and get back on track after a slip-up.

8.1 Structure and Content

Session 2 introduces regular eating, a key procedure of CBT for BED. The priorities of Session 2 are the following:

1. Reviewing and reinforcing real-time monitoring
2. Introducing regular eating

R. Dalle Grave et al., *Cognitive Behavior Therapy for Binge Eating Disorder*, https://doi.org/10.1007/978-3-031-71456-6_8

The session is structured as follows (the approximate duration of each element is shown in parentheses):

1. Reviewing the content of real-time monitoring (10–15 minutes).
2. Collaboratively setting the agenda for the session (2 minutes)
3. Working through the agenda and agreeing on homework tasks (up to 30 minutes)
4. Summarizing the session, confirming the homework assignments, and arranging the next appointment

We recommend adhering to this structure because failure to do so increases the risk of not addressing the patient's problems and therefore failure to implement key treatment procedures. The therapist should only deviate from this structure when adhering to it is impossible or seems inadequate (e.g., the patient is facing a severe interpersonal crisis or recent bereavement).

8.2 Reviewing the Content of Real-Time Self-Monitoring

Whereas in Session 1, the review of the monitoring records was focused on the *process* of monitoring, from Session 2 onwards, the review is mainly focused on its *content*. A review of the content of the monitoring records, if done well, calmly, and actively involving the patient, is of great help in shedding light on the processes maintaining the patient's eating disorder, and allows their personal formulation to be updated or amend. The therapist should assess whether each day is typical or atypical (and if so, in what way) and whether any features not yet included in the personal formulation emerge from the review. In the example below, the therapist reviews a patient's monitoring record (presented in Fig. 8.1).

Therapist: (*assessing Process #1, skipping breakfast*) I see that you didn't eat breakfast because you felt full. Can you explain to me what you mean by feeling full?

Patient: Er… that there was no room in my stomach.

Therapist: Is there a reason why you felt full?

Patient: I ate a lot the night before!

Therapist: Ah… Why? Did you lose control over your eating?

Patient: Yes.

Therapist: Okay. Would you have eaten breakfast if you hadn't lost control and felt so full?

Patient: Erm… Generally, I try to have a very light breakfast so I won't eat too much overall if I lose control during the day.

Therapist: What do you mean by light (*the therapist looks at other monitoring records to see what the patient has for breakfast on the other days*)?

Patient: I only have coffee.

Therapist: (*exploring Process #2*) I see that you had another coffee at work.

Patient: Yes.

Therapist: Don't you ever have a snack?

Date *18 March* Day *Wednesday*

Time	Food and drink consumed	Place	*	Comments
7:00	*1 coffee*	*Kitchen*		*I'll skip breakfast: I'm full* **(1)**
10:00	*1 coffee*	*Work bar*		**(2)**
13:00	*1 plate of pasta with tuna* *1 packet of breadsticks* *1 plate of mixed vegetables seasoned with oil and vinegar* *2 glasses of water* *1 apple*	*Office canteen*		
18:00	*1 packet of crisps* *30 biscuits* *10 shelled walnuts* *2 ice creams* *1 can of cola*	*Kitchen*	* * * * *	*Felt tired and sad* **(3)**
				I skipped dinner. I felt full and disgusted by what I ate. Tomorrow I'll skip breakfast and I'll just eat a salad for lunch.
22:00	*6 chocolates*		*	**(4)**

Daily steps	Number: *6,000* **(5)**	
Formal exercise	Type:	Duration (min):

Fig. 8.1 Example of a patient's monitoring record. (The numbers in parentheses are the processes investigated by the therapist and described in the text)

Patient: No, I'm not very hungry when I work.
Therapist: (*investigating Process #3*) You put a chain of asterisks at 6:00 p.m.
Patient: Yes, as usual, when I got home from work, I felt tired and sad, and I binged.
Therapist: Why did you start eating if you felt tired and sad?
Patient: Food makes me feel better… It's gratifying and makes me less sad.
Therapist: (*investigating Process #4 at 10:00 p.m.*) I see that you put an asterisk here.
Patient: Yes.
Therapist: So, it wasn't your intention to eat something?
Patient: No.
Therapist: Since it wasn't your intention, what made you start eating?

Patient: I don't know how to control myself. I'm not determined enough. I don't have enough willpower.

Therapist: (*investigating Process #5*) Do you know how many daily steps you usually took before starting this program?

Patient: I walked about 3000 steps a day.

Therapist: Congratulations, you have doubled your daily step number. That is a good start!

Patient: Thank you, it was not so difficult.

Reviewing the content of monitoring records requires specific skills since, as we have experienced during our training and supervision, some therapists tend to be prescriptive, indicating instead of eliciting the relationship between the various maintenance processes and/or suggesting patients make behavioural changes before understanding their usefulness. Here are some examples of prescriptive phrases that are not useful in a self-monitoring review: "*That binge-eating episode happened because you skipped lunch*", or "*If you had eaten more at lunch, you would have had a lower risk of binging*", *or* "*I see that you did not eat carbs at lunch. You should eat some rice so you will not binge later.*"

To help avoid such pitfalls, we suggest placing the patient's personal formulation next to their monitoring records, and to remember to ask questions rather than make statements. For example, the patient may be asked if the content of their monitoring records indicates any of the maintenance processes of the binge-eating episodes reported in their formulation. Once the patient comes to the realization that some features of their eating disorders (e.g., delaying eating) maintain their binge episodes, they will be more willing to address them.

8.3 Introducing Regular Eating

8.3.1 Rationale

The regular eating procedure is essential for the success of CBT for BED, and is considered the foundation on which other changes are built, and patients greatly value it. The focus is the patient's eating patterns, i.e., when they eat, rather than what or how much to eat. The goal is to help patients eat at regular intervals throughout the day.

If done well, the procedure rapidly reduces the frequency of binge-eating episodes and, at the end of Step One, most patients report only "residual" binge-eating episodes to be addressed during Step Two. The reduction in the frequency of binge-eating episodes is very reassuring and empowering for the patient, and is generally accompanied by a marked improvement in mood and self-efficacy. In addition, in patients with unstructured and chaotic eating habits (e.g., munching continuously throughout the day and not eating regular meals or snacks), the regular eating procedure provides them with structure and control.

Regular eating has two main positive effects [1]:

1. It tackles the tendency to delay eating, a form of dieting that is common among patients with binge eating.
2. After a few weeks, it generally reduces the frequency of binge-eating episodes and the degree of preoccupation with food and eating.

The regular eating procedure is introduced in Session 2, and this is the first time the patients are asked to change how they eat. For the explanation of the rationale behind the procedure, the therapist should refer to the patient's monitoring records to see if there a relationship between irregular eating and binge-eating episodes is apparent. Otherwise, the therapist might pragmatically say, "*It's time to start making the first changes to your eating habits. The goal is simply to eat regularly, not to alter the amount or type of food you eat. Eating regularly throughout the day is a great help for people with binge-eating episodes. Doing this, and doing it well, is very important, as it is the foundation upon which all other changes will be built.*"

8.3.2 Procedure

The regular eating procedure has two components [1]:

1. *Eating at regular intervals throughout the day*. This pattern involves eating three planned meals plus two or three planned snacks daily. For example:
   - Breakfast
   - Snack
   - Lunch
   - Snack
   - Evening meal
   - Evening snack (if appropriate)
2. *Not eating between planned meals and snacks*

8.3.3 Planning Ahead

The therapist should emphasize the importance of planning ahead to avoid being influenced by long-established eating habits that may have become automatic. *Planning should be done the night before (best solution) or, at the latest, on the morning of the same day*. The patient is invited to write in the first three columns of their monitoring record (i) when (in the "Time" column), (ii) what (in the "Food and drink consumed" column), and (iii) where (in the "Place" column) they will eat their meals and snacks. To emphasize the importance of planning ahead, the therapist can say, "*Planning is essential for all the reasons I just listed. Good planning means that if I call you at any time of the day, you should be able to tell me when and where you will eat your next meal, and what you are going to have. Of course, I won't do that, but you must understand what it means to plan ahead.*" If the next day's meal plan is unpredictable due a social occasion (e.g., lunch at a relative's or a birthday party at a friend's house), the patient should be encouraged to plan before starting the meal, having seen what food is available and found a private place to write down what to eat.

The therapist should suggest the patient allow a *maximum interval of 4 hours between meals and snacks*, informing them about the possible negative consequences of delayed eating or skipping a snack or a meal (e.g., increased risk of having a binge-eating episode).

The patient is asked to use a watch to ensure that they *eat when it is time,* i.e., according to the planned schedule. They should eat mindfully, observing their behaviour during meals without being influenced by external (e.g., the sight of food or environmental situations) or internal (e.g., food cravings, thoughts, or emotional changes) stimuli, which favour the intake of food that has not been planned. The therapist should explain that these feelings are altered by eating habits that have been operating for some time. To support this information, we use the example of travellers who move from one time zone to another. To adapt to the new time, the plan is to wake up when the day begins, sleep when it ends, and eat at set times appropriate for where they are, not where they have come from. Even when the patient has restored normal feelings of hunger and satiety as a result of regular eating, if indicated, it is advisable for them to do as most people do and not rely only on bodily sensations to decide when to eat. The therapist should also emphasize the importance of regular eating regardless of the circumstances, and that the eating plan can be easily adjusted to fit daily commitments (e.g., work activities).

If the patient asks for advice on what to eat, it should be reiterated that at this time, what or how much to eat is not important: the focus is on *when* to eat. Suppose, however, they insist on having advice on what to eat. In that case, the therapist can suggest adopting a varied eating plan with a minimum of avoided foods, and average portions that can be determined by recipes or the eating habits of friends or family.

Accepting the patient's definition of what constitutes a "meal" or "snack" is recommended, as long as they eat something. It is helpful to tell the patient to use common sense, so a soup may be accepted as a meal, but a cappuccino would be inadequate. In patients with very chaotic eating habits, however, regular eating may be introduced gradually. In such cases, we advise the patient to focus on the first part of the day, which is generally less problematic, and then, when there is an improvement in that part of the day, to move on to the second part.

When the therapist has finished explaining regular eating, it is helpful for them to give the patient a handout summarizing it to help them remember the key aspects of the procedure (see Table 8.1). The introduction of the regular eating procedure is a skill that all therapists using CBT for BED need to acquire. In this case too, its success or failure will be heavily influenced by the therapist's ability to convey the rationale well, addressing all objections and obstacles as they arise. Some patients adopt the procedure quickly, while others take three or more weeks. It is essential that regular eating and the difficulties encountered in applying this procedure are a constant topic of the sessions in Step One and sometimes in the subsequent phases of the treatment, and that all signs of progress are praised.

Table 8.1 The main features of regular eating

Eating regularly every 3–4 hours and not eating between meals is the foundation for further changes. The benefits of regular eating are to structure eating habits and the day, to address one of the three forms of dysfunctional dieting (skipping meals, the other two being eliminating foods and reducing portions), and to interrupt the cycle of alternating binge-eating episodes and dietary restraint.
To eat regularly, you need to adopt two behaviours:
1. *Eating three meals plus two snacks at regular, planned intervals* (every 3–4 hours), specifically:
8 a.m. breakfast
11 a.m. mid-morning snack
1 p.m. lunch
4 p.m. mid-afternoon snack
8 p.m. dinner
2. *Not eating between meals and snacks*
Points to keep in mind:
Eat your planned meals and snacks, but don't eat between meals.
Don't skip planned meals or snacks.
Don't let more than 4 hours go by without eating.
Always know when, where, and what to eat at your next meal or snack.

If some unforeseen event prevents you from eating at the set times, try to be flexible and not too rigid to better adapt to the situation. Adapting to these unforeseen events will allow you to manage the various situations that require changing the usual mealtime (e.g., work, holidays, invitations to dinner, etc.).

8.3.4 Self-Monitoring in Real Time

Patients should be encouraged to put their monitoring record, on which they have written planned meals and snacks, on the table beside them while they eat. This will enable them to record the relevant behaviours, thoughts, emotions, and events "in the moment" at which they are experienced, using the procedure described in Sect. 6.5. The therapist should explain to the patient that continuing real-time monitoring will help them adhere to meal planning, and make it easier for them to interrupt behaviours that seem automatic and out of control. Figure 8.2 shows the monitoring record of a patient who implemented the regular eating procedure, planning when, what, and where to eat at the top of the monitoring record and, below the line, their monitoring in real time.

8.3.5 Things to Say and Do

This procedure is used to help the patient eat when and what they planned if they get into difficulties. The therapist should specify that it is essential to pay attention to this aspect of the regular eating procedure, not so much because of the effect it could

Date *19 April* Day *Thursday*

Time	Food and drink consumed	Place	*	Comments
	Today's Plan			
7 am	*1 coffee* *1 pot of low-fat yoghurt* *2 oatcakes with jam*	*Home, kitchen*		
10 am	*1 apple*	*Office*		
1 pm	*1 plate of pasta with tomato sauce and 1 teaspoon of parmesan cheese* *1 serving of raw vegetables drizzled with a little olive oil*	*Office canteen*		
4:30 pm	*1 packet of crackers* *1 banana*	*Office*		
8 pm	*1 pot of low-fat yoghurt* *2 slices of chicken breast* *1 portion of potatoes* *1 serving of boiled carrots* *1 apple*	*Home, kitchen*		
				All ok. Istuck to the plan.
7 am	*1 coffee* *1 pot of low-fat yoghurt* *2 oatcakes with jam*	*Home, kitchen*		
10 am	*1 apple*	*Office*		
1 pm	*1 plate of pasta with tomato sauce* *1 teaspoon Parmesan cheese* *1 serving of raw vegetables drizzled with a little olive oil* *1 packet of crackers* *1 orange*	*Office canteen*		*There were no bananas so I hadan orange*
4:30 pm	*1 pot of low-fat yoghurt*	*Office*		
8 pm	*2 slices of chicken breast* *1 portion of potatoes* *1 serving of boiled carrots* *1 apple*	*Home, kitchen*		
10 pm				*I had a strong craving for chocolate ,but I told myself I could tolerateit and didn't eat any. I'm satisfied with how the day went, it's the first day inmonths that I haven't binged*

Fig. 8.2 An example of a monitoring record showing implementation of the regular eating procedure

have on their body weight (many people may sporadically eat between meals or eat more per meal without this changing their weight), but because of the negative consequences that deviations can have on eating concerns (e.g., increasing worry about overeating) and behaviour (e.g., the reaction to breaking a dietary rule can lead to a binge-eating episode or skipping the next meal). After this premise, the therapist should explain to the patient why and how to implement the "things to say and do" procedure, and ask them to apply it as early as the following week. "Things to say" are personal mottos that will help them to "urge-surf", i.e., resist the urge until it diminishes, and "things to do" are activities that will take their mind off the urge, to put it off for a while. The steps of the procedure are as follows [2].

- Preparing a "coping card" (an index card, Post-it, or note on their smartphone) with written "things to say and do" to consult when they perceive the urge to deviate from their meal plan.
- When the urge strikes, getting out the coping card and analyzing the list of things to say and do, going through them individually and choosing the strategy(s) that seems most appropriate for the circumstance.
- In real time, writing in the Comments column of the monitoring record which strategy would best help them avoid deviating from the plan.

For the procedure to work, it is essential that the patient learns to recognize the urge to deviate from the plan as soon as possible, that they apply the procedure immediately (those who hesitate are lost!), and that they fill out the monitoring record in real time.

Things to say (also known as the "urge surfing" strategy) should be phrases that make it easier to tolerate the urge to eat by deviating from planning (e.g., "I can tolerate this urge for food without eating; the urge increases until it reaches a peak, then recedes and vanishes, like a wave."). Things to do (also known as "alternative activities") should be distracting, preferably enjoyable activities that take at least an hour. Possible activities are the following [3]:

- Interpersonal activities (e.g., chatting or hanging out with friends)
- Getting out of the situation (e.g., going for a walk)
- Changing the mood (e.g., listening to music incompatible with the binge-eating episode).

Table 8.2 provides some example of things to say and things to do.

Table 8.2 Example of things to say and do to avert the urge to deviate from regular eating

Things to Say
This craving for food is fleeting, and I can resist it
I can withstand it
The craving for food is a wave; if I let some time pass, I won't feel it anymore
If I hold on, then I know it'll get better
It's hard, but I can do it!
Things to Do
Take a hot shower
Brush my teeth
Call a friend
Message with a friend
Go to a friend's house
Go out for a walk
Listen to my favourite music

8.3.6 Reducing Food Stimuli

Environmental stimuli, such as the presence at home of large amounts of palatable food, promote unregulated and excessive eating and binge-eating episodes. It is, therefore, essential to educate the patient to adopt strategies that reduce their exposure to excessive environmental food stimuli, and thus facilitate their adherence to regular eating. To this end, we give the patient an exhaustive list of strategies to reduce temptation, as shown in Table 8.3. The list was designed to include several everyday situations in which people typically encounter environmental food stimuli, which may trigger binge-eating episodes. After examining the environmental stimuli relevant to the patient, we discuss possible ways to reduce them and agree on specific homework tasks.

8.3.7 Getting Back on Track

Patients should be advised that learning the procedure for regular eating and applying it takes time. It is almost inevitable to slip up during this process of changing eating habits (e.g., skipping a meal or snack, sometimes eating less or more than planned, or having an episode of binge eating). The patient should be educated that when this occurs, it is essential to get back on track immediately, not to wait until the next day. They should try to understand what triggered their loss of control, and fight the all-or-nothing attitude (either perfect control over eating or no control at all). They should not consider the day as a single unit (with the entire day being lost if something goes wrong).

Table 8.3 Environmental stimuli that hinder weight loss, and strategies to mitigate them

Shopping for groceries
Plan in detail what to buy (i.e., based on weekly meal planning).
Only shop on a full stomach.
Shop according to a list, and don't buy food you don't need.
Don't take more money than you need.
Avoid the dessert counter and the highly tempting shops.
Buy food that requires preparation.
Storing food
Don't leave food in sight.
Store food supplies only in the kitchen or pantry.
Store food in set places.
Store food covered with foil or in opaque containers.
Put tempting foods in inaccessible places.
Preparing food
Cook the exact amount of food and prepare individual portions.
Cook with as little fat or oil as possible.
Don't taste food during its preparation.
Don't cook when you're hungry.
Chew gum while cooking.
Soak dishes and utensils that you have just used for cooking in soapy water.
Serving food
Serve food on individual plates rather than platters.
Avoid putting a breadbasket on the table.
Wait 5 minutes between courses.
Use small plates.
While eating
Take small bites and chew for a long time.
Put your cutlery down between mouthfuls.
Always eat in the same place.
Always eat seated at the table.
Focus on what you eat.
Focus on the taste of food.
Eat at precise times every day.
Eat according to your meal plan and not based on feelings of hunger or temptation.
After Eating
Get up from the table immediately after finishing your meal.
Clear the table immediately after you have finished eating.
If possible, move away from the kitchen.
Drink coffee in the living room.
Don't store too many leftovers.
Wrap leftover food in foil.

8.4 Summarizing the Session, Setting the Homework, and Arranging the Next Appointment

At the end of Session 2, the following homework is typically agreed upon with patients: (i) continuing real-time self-monitoring, (ii) resisting weighing at home, and (iii) starting regular eating. The therapist should end the session by summarizing its content, repeating the homework assignments, and setting the date and time of the next appointment.

References

1. Fairburn CG. Cognitive behavior therapy and eating disorders. New York: Guilford Press; 2008.
2. Dalle Grave R, Sartirana M, El Ghoch M, Calugi S. Treating obesity with personalized cognitive behavioral therapy. Cham: Springer; 2018.
3. Dalle Grave R, Calugi S. Cognitive behavior therapy for adolescents with eating disorders. New York: Guilord Press; 2020.

Implementing the Rest of Step One

9

Abstract

The remaining five sessions of Step One are principally focused on assessing the patient's progress in not weighing between sessions, adopting an active lifestyle, and implementing regular eating. Another new procedure to address the patient's eating style is introduced if it is contributing to dysregulated eating and overeating. Patients are advised to formalize eating, consuming meals with clear beginnings and ends, seated at the table. Other suggestions are avoiding eating directly from packages or pans, not associating eating with other activities, addressing "grazing" or "picking at" food, and abnormal eating speeds

Having completed the first three sessions of Step One, the patient should now:

- Be reasonably well engaged in treatment
- Have understood and accepted the personal formulation
- Be adept at monitoring in real time
- Have accepted weekly in-session collaborative weighing
- Have started to increase their physical activity level
- Have begun regular eating

This chapter describes the remaining procedures of Step One (i.e., sessions 4–7).

R. Dalle Grave et al., *Cognitive Behavior Therapy for Binge Eating Disorder*,
https://doi.org/10.1007/978-3-031-71456-6_9

9.1 Structure

The priority from Session 4 onwards is to evaluate the patient's progress in not weighing between sessions, adopting an active lifestyle, and implementing regular eating. Another new procedure to introduce is addressing the style of eating.

9.2 Addressing Weighing Between Sessions

A few patients find it particularly challenging to resist the urge to weigh themselves between sessions, and lapses in this regard may, therefore, occur. As described in Chap. 6, frequent weighing increases weight concerns because of fluctuating but insignificant changes in hydration status. Increases in weight concern, in turn, may lead to either accentuation of dysfunctional dietary restraint or, at the opposite end of the scale, temporary abandonment of eating control. If the patient reports a tendency to weigh themselves between sessions, the therapist should address this dysfunctional behaviour in a manner similar to that described in the following transcript.

Therapist: (*reading the comments column on the patient's monitoring record*) I see you have weighed yourself between sessions.

Patient: Yes, I'm sorry… I shouldn't have… I couldn't stop myself from doing it!

Therapist: Don't be sorry. We knew that it could happen. That's why I asked you to write the number on the scales every time you weigh yourself between sessions, and to describe the events, thoughts and emotions associated with this behaviour in the Comments column. I see, however, that you did weigh yourself most days before starting this programme. You did it every day, even several times a day.

Patient: Yes, that's true!

Therapist: I know it's difficult to resist the urge to weigh yourself. I see that you have reported on your monitoring record for Tuesday that your weight was 85 kg four days after our in-session collaborative weighing. Why did you check your weight on Tuesday rather than waiting for the next session, only three days later?

Patient: I wanted to see if I was putting on weight!

Therapist: What did you conclude after seeing that number on the scales?

Patient: I'd put on half a kilo

Therapist: So, did weighing yourself have a positive or negative effect?

Patient: I was a little demoralized!

Therapist: Did you do anything to manage your demoralization?

Patient: I skipped my snack.

Therapist: Yes, I see from your monitoring record that you had planned to eat a snack, but you skipped it. I also see that you put some asterisks after dinner.

Patient: I ate a box of cookies I didn't plan on!

Therapist: What prompted you to eat cookies?

Patient: I was upset.

Therapist: What made you feel upset? Did it have anything to do with the weight you saw earlier in the day?

Patient: Well, yes, I was upset because I have been eating regularly, but I had put on weight anyway!

Therapist: Were you upset even though you had skipped a snack?

Patient: Yes, I'm always afraid that what I've done isn't enough!

Therapist: So, tell me if I have understood correctly. You checked your weight to see if you were gaining weight, and you found that the number on the scales had increased by half a kilo. So, you got upset and skipped a snack as a reaction to supposedly having put on weight. However, despite this dietary restriction, you continued to feel upset, and then ate some biscuits to make yourself feel less upset.

Patient: Yes, it seems it happened exactly like that!

Therapist: It appears to me that weighing yourself between sessions led you to binge for two reasons. I can see two mechanisms acting here (*indicates patient's personal formulation*): the first relates to your interpretation of the number on the scales, which prompted you to skip a snack and, therefore, binge in the evening because you were hungrier, and the second concerns the demoralization associated with the confirmation of your doubts that you were gaining weight.

Patient: Indeed!

Therapist: If I can give an example, it's like an entrepreneur who is very afraid of his company going bankrupt, and for this reason, looks at the sales figures daily. Seeing that they have not increased in one day, she begins to get worried and decides to take action to increase sales by launching an advertising campaign. However, this costs money, and causes an economic loss. By spending money without waiting to get a comprehensive vision of her sales overall, she made her pessimistic prophecies come true.

Patient: Yes! So, I have to resist not weighing myself all week, no matter how worried I am!

Therapist: Yes, I think it would be best for you to resist the urge to weigh yourself, and instead focus more on eating regularly. I'm convinced that that will be more helpful in managing your weight and binging in the long run. Remember also that it is impossible to interpret a single reading on the scales, as any short-term weight change is due to alterations in the water content in your body.

Patient: Okay, I'll try not to weigh myself between sessions!

9.3 Addressing Obstacles to Adopting an Active Lifestyle

The therapist should empathetically investigate (rather than speculate on) the patient's obstacles to increasing their physical activity levels. In general, many obstacles reported by our patients include lack of motivation and low perceived self-efficacy, no history of fitness training, lack of ability to cope, and environmental and socioeconomic barriers such as inadequate access to gyms or other facilities, high cost of training programmes, low social and cultural support, and time constraints [1]. Other obstacles more specific to individuals with BED and clinical obesity (see Sect. 4.3.1 and Table 4.4 for the definition) include low fitness levels, physical conditions (e.g., arthritis, obstructive sleep apnoea), boredom and lack of stimulation, lethargy, unfavourable comparisons with others, shame associated with body exposure, embarrassment, and fear of injury or death. Clinical depression, often associated with BED, is an additional and important obstacle to exercise.

Once the individual obstacles have been identified, the next step is to discuss with the patient their motivations for and against doing exercise. It is best to start by asking the patient to list the negative aspects of change: whether a sedentary lifestyle offers them any perceived benefits that they fear or begrudge missing out on. Subsequently, the patient should be asked to weigh the benefits. At this stage, we encourage the patient to reflect on the short- and long-term effects of exercise on their physical and psychological quality of life and ability to control their weight. To have a handy reference for the future, the list of pros and cons should be written down as a "pros and cons of change" table, as that desctibed in Chap. 7 (Table 7.1). The goal is to help the patient conclude that exercise will be necessary for them to be able to control their eating and weight in the long term and reduce the medical and psychosocial complications associated with clinical obesity. As such, every reason for change must be reinforced, and all negative aspects of change addressed.

Hence, the next step is to think collaboratively with the patient about how to address the obstacles to exercise they have identified. If there are serious physical barriers (e.g., severe orthopaedic, cardiac, or pulmonary diseases), the type of physical exercise to do and the obstacles to address should be discussed with the doctor managing the comorbid conditions. In all other cases we address obstacles using the proactive problem-solving procedure described in Chap. 13. We also educate the patient that, at first, doing physical activity will be hard, but it will gradually become more pleasurable. As dysfunctional thoughts may represent an obstacle to adopting an active lifestyle, it is helpful to assist the patient in identifying any they may have and replacing them with more functional thoughts (see Table 9.1)

Table 9.1 Dysfunctional thoughts creating an obstacle to increasing physical activity levels and alternative functional thoughts

Dysfunctional thought	Functional thought
After a day of work, I am too tired to do physical activity	*The fatigue accumulated during the day is mainly due to nervous tension, and physical activity helps reduce stress fatigue. A walk will help me feel better and less stressed.*
I don't have time	*I can find 20–30 minutes to dedicate to the physical activity*
I'm too fat	*Physical activity is the best way to control body weight and keep fit*
There is no one to take care of the children for me	*I can take a walk with my children or get a babysitter for the hours I dedicate to physical activity; the money spent will not be thrown away, because it will be invested in improving my health*
I'm too old	*Walking is a physical exercise suitable for all ages. Regular physical activity will help slow down my ageing process*
I'm too depressed	*Physical activity helps to improve mood and manage depression*

It can also be helpful to suggest that patients create some incentives to maintaining an active lifestyle. Here are some examples:

- Buying sportswear
- Planning physical activity (what, where, when, and for how long)
- Preparing workout clothes the night before and putting them where they are visible on waking
- Keeping a workout bag in the car so it is always to hand
- Setting an alarm as a reminder that it's time to exercise
- Arranging exercise dates with friends
- Calling friends to remind them of their exercise dates
- Rewarding oneself after having done the planned physical activity

9.4 Addressing Obstacles to Regular Eating

Below are the most common difficulties reported by our patients in eating regularly and how we address them.

Knowing in advance what I'm eating increases my preoccupation with eating. I want to be more spontaneous.

In this case, the therapist should ask the patient if they feel genuinely spontaneous at this time. It may be helpful, taking an example from a patient's monitoring record, to analyze whether the regularity of meals and snacks has been conditioned by their eating concern, pointing out that perhaps being spontaneous at this point in therapy might be unrealistic and premature. The therapist should encourage the patient to try out or persevere with the procedure by emphasizing that it is designed to help them avoid being influenced by dietary concerns and dysfunctional eating habits. In addition, they should also reiterate that the regular eating procedure is temporary and will allow them not only to reduce the frequency of binge-eating episodes but also to gather information on the relationship between eating and weight, which can reduce both weight and eating concerns. It is also useful to reassure the patient that therapy aims to help them become more spontaneous and free in their eating, but this will only happen when their binge-eating episodes are reduced. Just like you need to know the grammatical rules of a foreign language by heart before you can converse freely in it.

Planning doesn't work. I binge when I don't stick to the meal plan.

This objection refers to the common tendency of patients to interpret even the slightest deviations from the eating plan as "a failure", and to consider the whole day ruined. Such a reaction is a typical example of all-or-nothing thinking, in which any outcome other than perfect adherence is considered grounds for abandoning the plan entirely. To help a patient cope with this reaction, the therapist should explain the phenomenon, educate them about this dysfunctional way of interpreting events, and then explain to them that there are different degrees of adherence to regular eating. To demonstrate this, the therapist and the patient could look at their monitoring record and give each day over the previous week a score of 0–5 (five being the number of meals and snacks planned) on their degree of adherence to regular eating.

Eating mid-morning and mid-afternoon snacks will make me put on weight.

In this case, the therapist should validate the patient's concern and reassure them that, however, this outcome rarely occurs because the goal is not to change the amount of food they are eating. In addition, regular eating will reduce the frequency of binge-eating episodes and, consequently, the total energy intake. Despite these reassurances and explanations, the patient may tend to eat low-energy snacks, but the therapist should not object to this choice because, at this stage of treatment, it is important *when* they eat, not what or how much.

Things to say and things to do are useless because they only delay a binge-eating episode.

To address this objection, the therapist may explain that the point of the "things to say and do" procedure is for them to develop skills to manage the urge to eat between meals and snacks, and that this is a crucial step towards recovery from the eating disorder. In addition, even if the urge to eat returns after an hour or two, this does not negate the success of managing the previous urge: the goal is to learn to overcome the urge to eat for a few hours (i.e., the time between meals from snacks). As with all new skills, it will require practice.

I've never eaten this way, and none of my family or friends eat this way.

In this case, the therapist should respond that regular eating will help them overcome the eating disorder and provide the foundation for other changes. Once the disorder is in remission, it will be up to them to decide how to eat, but it is advisable to eat this way for now. It should be noted, however, that this is a healthy way to eat from a physiological point of view. Some patients are reluctant to eat breakfast, fearing that if they start their day eating, they will not be able to stop. Regular eating is an opportunity to test and refute these dysfunctional beliefs.

We also encourage patients to apply the procedures described in Chap. 8 to facilitate adherence to the regular eating procedure (i.e., planning ahead, self-monitoring in real time, using alternative activities and urge surfing, reducing the environmental food stimuli and getting back on track).

9.5 Addressing Eating Style

It is not usually necessary to address the patient's eating style unless it is contributing to their dysregulated eating and overeating. Below are some indications we give to our patients who report this problem [2, 3]:

- *Formalized eating*. We recommend that it is best that meals have a clear beginning and end, and meals at home should only be eaten when seated at a set place.
- *Avoiding eating directly from packages or pans*. We suggest preparing meals and taking them to the dining table. Furthermore, any remaining food should be cleared away before eating. The availability of easy-access and/or tempting food not requiring any preparation should be limited at this point until control over eating has been regained.
- *Not associating eating with other activities*. It is easy to overeat while doing activities such as messaging, surfing the net, using social media, reading, or watching television. For this reason, we suggest to patients not to do anything else while eating. Eating consciously and enjoying food will help them to adhere to what they have planned, and avoid overeating.
- *Addressing "grazing" or "picking at" food*. If patients have a habit of munching on food between meals or snacks or when they are preparing a meal, this may destabilize their attempts to stick to a pattern of regular eating. If this is an issue, we suggest applying the "things to say and do" procedure (see Chap. 8).
- *Abnormal eating speeds*. "Wolfing" is a behaviour typical of binge eating and should not be considered an issue, as the goal is for patients to stop binge eating entirely rather than change how they do it. However, rapid eating when not binging may result in overeating, and patients who display this behaviour should be encouraged to moderate their eating speed, as slowing down generally helps them control how much they eat. Strategies for slowing eating suggested to these

patients include taking sips of water or putting cutlery down between bites, engaging in conversation at the table, and mimicking the eating speed of fellow diners. Other tips can be found in Table 8.3.

References

1. Sherwood NE, Jeffery RW. The behavioral determinants of exercise: implications for physical activity interventions. Annu Rev Nutr. 2000;20:21–44. https://doi.org/10.1146/annurev.nutr.20.1.21.
2. Fairburn CG. Cognitive behavior therapy and eating disorders. New York: Guilford Press; 2008.
3. Dalle Grave R, Calugi S. Cognitive behavior therapy for adolescents with eating disorders. New York: Guilford Press; 2020.

Involving Significant Others

10

Abstract

Cognitive behaviour thearpy (CBT) for binge-eating disorder BED is an individual treatment. However, the significant others of adult patients (whether friends, partners, or parents) are involved in some joint sessions if they may facilitate treatment and the patient agrees to their assistance (generally in about one-third of adult cases). Three to four joint sessions may be held after individual ones, and the goal is to recruit significant others to help create an optimal environment to facilitate patient change. With adolescent patients, parents are always involved, given the age and circumstances of these patients. Parental involvement is usually limited to one short joint session with the patient at the end of the individual assessment/preparation phase, one with parents alone in the first week of treatment, and as many joint sessions at the end of a patient's individual session as required. These joint sessions, in both adolescents and adults, should last about 15 minutes.

10.1 Adult Patients

CBT for adults with BED is an individual treatment. Still, significant others (i.e., friends, partners, or parents) may be involved if it appears that they might facilitate treatment, provided that the patient agrees to their involvement [1]. The goal of recruiting significant others is for them to help create an optimal environment for change. Typically, three to four joint sessions with significant others of about 15 minutes each immediately after individual sessions are scheduled. Generally, we plan joint sessions in nearly one-third of our patients.

The two specific indications that we adopt for including significant others are the following: (i) if it seems like they can help the patient to make changes; (ii) if they appear to be hindering attempts by the patient to change (e.g., buying too much unhealthy food or making negative comments about their behaviour and/or weight).

R. Dalle Grave et al., *Cognitive Behavior Therapy for Binge Eating Disorder*, https://doi.org/10.1007/978-3-031-71456-6_10

In some cases, another potential benefit is to dispel the secrecy about binge-eating episodes. Indeed, some patients with BED maintain the secret of their eating problem for years, and this contributes to the maintenance of binge-eating episodes. When a patient shares their problematic eating behaviour with significant others, they can no longer fall back on secrecy and are, therefore, incentivised to engage in the treatment. Furthermore, in most cases, family and friends are generally supportive rather than critical, expediating the patient's attempt to change.

If the patient agrees to the involvement of significant others, the joint sessions must be prepared well in advance. The therapist should outline the objectives and content of these sessions to the patient, explaining that they will be focused on discussing how their family member or housemate, etc., can create a home environment that will facilitate their attempt to change their eating habits. It is important to underline that no topics beyond the objective of the treatment will be discussed.

Generally, the first joint session is scheduled after the patient has been in treatment for 2–3 weeks. It begins with an introduction by the therapist and an explanation of its purpose. The patient is then asked to explain the nature of the treatment, all the positive changes in eating and physical activity they have achieved up to that point, and the obstacles they would like help to address.

The next step is for both the patient and the therapist to listen to the points of view expressed by significant others, providing answers to any questions they may have. Common questions are whether it would be helpful for them to comment on or check the food the patient is eating, and how they might best encourage them to follow the eating and physical activity plan. All questions should be addressed in the same session, with the therapist encouraging the patient to openly express what type of help they wish to receive from their significant others. While some patients prefer receiving support and advice on what to eat and encouragement to exercise, others perceive comments on eating and physical activity as criticism, and prefer that significant others refrain from making such comments.

Based on this information, the next part of the joint session will be a discussion of what precisely a significant other may do to help the patient. Overall, support that patients may like to receive from significant others can be divided into two main categories:

1. *Creating an optimal home environment.* The goal is to create a home environment that will promote positive eating habits and changes in physical activity. Significant others can be involved in helping the patient to shop for groceries, planning in detail the food to buy, preparing and serving meals (see Table 8.3), and reinforcing positive eating behaviours. They are also encouraged to adopt a supportive attitude and accept any setbacks the patient might experience.
2. *Helping to implement some of the treatment procedures.* As the patient decides, significant others can help by doing physical activity and/or planning the meals and snacks together with them, reducing environmental food stimuli, and avoiding keeping junk food in the house.

Some family members are very critical of patients with BED and clinical obesity (see Sect. 4.3.1 and Table 4.4 for the definition) about their weight, eating, and physical activity levels. In such cases, it is important to address their critical communication style, since they can create negative emotions and reactions in the patient and, paradoxically, trigger behaviours opposite to those they expected (e.g., binge-eating episodes). In most cases, criticisms and weight stigma are based on a lack of knowledge of the causes of eating disorders and clinical obesity, conditions that people often believe are the individual's "fault", due to their greed, laziness, and/or lack of willpower [2]. Therefore, significant others need to be educated about the nature of BED and clinical obesity, and how they are considered and treated. In particular, the therapist should underline that they result from a complex interaction of genetic and environmental factors [3, 4]. Moreover, clinical obesity is a chronic medical disease, rather than a failing, that requires continuous care [5, 6]. At the same time, several psychological and behavioural mechanisms maintain dysfunctional eating and exercise habits. It is not merely a question of lack of willpower. To explain this concept, the therapist should describe the personal formulation of the patient and inform them of goals of the treatment. They should be very specific about the involvement of significant others in providing active and helpful support to patients, avoiding any form of criticism, because that would reduce their chances of success rather than fostering it.

10.2 Adolescent Patients

The same principles apply to the treatment of adolescent patients, except for the fact that parents are always involved, given the age and circumstances of these patients. Involving parents in CBT of adolescent patients with BED is recommended for the following reasons, among others [7]:

- Parents have the right and responsibility to make important decisions regarding the treatment of their teenage children, and treatment cannot be commenced without their informed consent.
- How parents react to the symptoms of the adolescent with a BED may influence the severity of their eating-disorder psychopathology [8], and positively or negatively affect the treatment outcome [9].
- As adolescents with eating disorders usually live with their parents, the latter can be of direct assistance in helping them to address the process of maintaining eating-disorder psychopathology or, in contrast, may be unwittingly hindering or preventing the change.

Parental involvement requires a slight adaptation of CBT for BED, as in most sessions the adolescent patient is seen alone. Parental involvement is usually limited to one short joint session with the patient at the end of the individual assessment and preparation phase, one with parents alone in the first week of treatment, and several more with the patient and therapist at the end of patients' individual sessions. As in adults, these joint sessions last about 15 minutes.

10.2.1 Joint Sessions during Assessment and Preparation

The first joint session aims to provide the parents with general information about their adolescent child's eating disorder, the nature of CBT-E, and the role that they should play in the treatment. We explain the cognitive behaviour model of BED maintenance, and how it interacts with clinical obesity (see Chap. 2). We also inform parents that while many adolescent patients recover completely from their eating disorder, and that there is no reason to think that this will not happen to their child, clinical obesity is a condition caused by a complex interaction of genetic and environmental factors that can be managed, but from which one cannot recover.

Then, we describe CBT for BED, underlining that the first 4 weeks of the treatment (i.e., Step One) will be mainly dedicated to helping their child understand the nature of their eating disorder and establishing a regular eating pattern to reduce the binge-eating episodes, not to lose weight. They will begin to address a reasonable and healthy weight loss only after establishing a regular eating pattern.

We also explain to parents that there are two approaches to treating eating disorders in adolescents. One is based on the medical model, in which external control (i.e., by parents, doctors, healthcare professionals) is required to overcome the problem, as the patients are considered not to be in control of their illness (the illness controls their behaviour). The other, which CBT adheres to, is based on the psychological model, which adopts a collaborative approach and never obliges patients to do something they do not want to do and do not see as a problem (they must learn to control their illness). We explain that the CBT approach is to first educate a patient, one-to-one, about their eating disorder and higher weight (if indicated) and the mechanisms that are maintaining it, which are then addressed through personalized specific strategies and procedures. Although it is the patient themself who will be implementing these strategies and procedures, parents will have an important role to play by creating a positive home environment that is likely to support the patient's efforts to change. They may also, in some cases, help their child to apply specific treatment procedures.

At the end of the first joint session, if parents agree to the proposal, it is suggested that they help their child weigh up the pros and cons of starting treatment. However, we emphasize that the decision to start the treatment will be made exclusively by their child, because the treatment will have no chance of success if a patient feels pressured by others into making this decision.

After the second assessment and preparation session, a second joint interview with the patient and the parents is held. If applicable, parents are informed that their child has decided to start treatment, and the nature and structure of CBT-E and the parent's role in the treatment are briefly reviewed.

10.2.2 Parents-Only Session

A single 50-minute session is scheduled with parents alone during the first week of Step One. Except for family crises, extreme difficulties during meals, or parental hostility towards the patient, this is usually the only parental session that the patient does not attend. The rationale behind and general content of the session is, however, explained to the young patient beforehand to maintain the trust that has already been built up between them and the therapist.

The main aim of the parents-only session is to identify and address potential family factors preventing or hindering the patient's attempts to change, and to suggest specific tips for creating an optimal family environment to facilitate the patient's efforts to change. The family environment is assessed in association with education about BED and higher weight (if indicated). The following areas should be explored [7]:

- The development and the current status of the patient's eating disorder. We ask parents about their perception of the eating disorder, its onset and evolution, and the resulting psychological, interpersonal, and school performance impairment. We also take a brief history of the medical and psychiatric history of both the adolescent and family, including any previous treatments for eating disorders and higher weight.
- The parents' knowledge about the causes of BED and body weight regulation. This can help to understand their comments and reactions to their child's eating habits and body weight.
- The parents' interpretation of and reactions to the patient's eating and body weight.
- The adolescent's reaction to the parents' behaviour and attitudes. For example, critical comments on eating and body weight may produce a change of mood, triggering a binge-eating episode or other dysfunctional behaviours.
- The presence in the home environment of factors that encourage overeating, dysfunctional dieting, and weight stigma. This assessment includes information about family eating styles and attitudes, the presence of family members with dysregulated eating and overeating, and those adopting extreme and inflexible dietary rules, or harbouring negative attitudes toward people with higher weight.

Regarding education, we present the cognitive behaviour theory of eating disorders and higher weight maintenance (see Chap. 2) to parents, together with their child's personal formulation (see Chap. 6 and Sect. 6.3) and how the treatment is structured (see Chap. 5). Then, we give parents the following general information on BED and their role in the treatment [7]:

- Parents have not caused their children's eating disorder, but their reactions can positively or negatively influence the recovery process.
- Parents may facilitate the recovery process by adopting the role of "helpers", rather than "controllers".
- Parents can create an optimal home environment that facilitates their child's effort to effect change.

We also give parents some specific advice, which can be divided into the following four categories [7]:

1. *On adopting a warm and functional communication style*. Dysfunctional communication between the parent and their child can adversely impact their child's mood. This may aggravate eating-disorder behaviours, as the adolescent may attempt to dispel their negative moods through unhealthy coping strategies (e.g., binge-eating episodes, self-harm, drug or alcohol misuse). It is, therefore, helpful for the parents to communicate with their child warmly, understandingly and calmly. This communication style signals that they understand their suffering and have empathy. Combining this with a positive attitude can instil hope in their ability to overcome their problems.
2. *On spending stress-free time with their child*. Time should be set aside for sharing pleasurable activities, reliving happy memories, and generally having fun together, away from the potential stresses of food, in a warm and loving atmosphere.
3. *On taking time for themselves and asking for support*. This involves having access to a support network (e.g., to have another family member available to step in) and dedicating time to self-care.
4. *On changing the home environment*. This involves avoiding following a strict diet and not keeping junk food in the house, making negative comments about the adolescent's eating during meals, or having conversations that emphasize thinness. It is also helpful to create an environment that does not encourage concerns about shape and weight, and to ensure that the teen is accessing a supportive, rather than harmful, digital environment.

Finally, any known barriers to change posed by parents should be addressed. Examples are disagreement between parents on treatment, parental clinical depression or other mental disorders, and pessimism on the utility of CBT due to previous treatment failure(s).

10.2.3 Joint Parent–Patient Sessions

The goals of the joint sessions with the patient and their parent during the treatment are (i) to inform parents of what is happening in the treatment and update them on the patient's progress, and (ii) to discuss how they might help the patient to implement certain treatment procedures. The frequency and number of these sessions, which are scheduled at the end of an individual session and last about 15 minutes, are flexible and should be decided based on the patient's individual needs. In most cases, however, the first joint parent–patient session is scheduled at the end of Session 3, after the regular eating procedure is introduced. This session should be dedicated to explaining to parents how they may help the patient implement it. This joint session will focus on the parents' role before, during, and after meals.

Parental involvement is often extremely helpful in helping the adolescent establish a regular eating pattern. After the therapist has explained the rationale behind and practical aspects of regular eating to the patient, and the patient has agreed to apply the procedure and that it would be helpful for their parents to be involved, the

Table 10.1 What parents can do to help their child implement regular eating

Leave the patient free to plan what to eat, but ensure that the kinds of food and drink the patient plans to eat are available.
Work with the patient to prepare joint meals following the written plan devised by the patient.
Encourage the patient to sit at the table if they are hesitant to eat at the planned time.
Try to eat most meals with the patient.
Avoid urging the patient to eat differently than planned.
Create a positive atmosphere by avoiding discussions about food, and arguments during meals.
Be supportive and not coercive. In difficult situations during meals, empathize and use supportive phrases (e.g., "We know that the process toward recovery is hard, but we are here to help you. Try to stick to your plan without being influenced by what you think or feel.").
Help the patient to practice distracting activities after eating to help them control the urge to resort to compensatory behaviours.

therapist should call the parents into the treatment room at the end of the session. In the presence of the patient, the therapist should provide the information previously discussed on the rationale behind and importance of the regular eating procedure. The parents should be told that the intervention is vital to the success of treatment, as it is the foundation upon which other changes are built. The positive effects of implementing regular eating, in particular the fact that it helps reduce the frequency of binge-eating episodes in adolescents, should be conveyed. The therapist should then explain that the procedure has two components: eating three planned meals each day, plus two or three planned snacks, and not eating between these set times. The focus at this stage of the treatment is to establish a pattern of regular eating, and therefore only *when* food is consumed is of concern.

The rest of the session should then be dedicated to discussing the parents' role in supporting the patient's efforts to eat regularly. The advice we usually offer about their behaviour around mealtimes is summarized in Table 10.1 [7]:

Other joint sessions are usually set up one week later, to refine the parents' help in implementing the regular eating procedure, and when with the patient with higher weight has collaboratively decided to work towards a reasonable and healthy weight loss. Finally, parents may be involved in helping the adolescent patient implement other CBT for BED procedures, as appropriate. As a general guideline, the therapist first explains the rationale behind and practical aspects of the procedure to the patient. Then, if they agree to implement them, the parents may be involved, provided that both the therapist and the patient think they may be able to facilitate its application.

References

1. Fairburn CG. Cognitive behavior therapy and eating disorders. New York: Guilford Press; 2008.
2. Phul RM. Stigma, discrimination, and obesity. In: Brownell KD, Walsh BT, editors. Eating disorders and obesity: a comprehensive handbook. 3rd ed. New York: Guilford Press; 2017. p. 134–9.

3. Citrome L. Binge eating disorder revisited: what's new, what's different, what's next – Addendum. CNS Spectr. 2019;24(S1):82. https://doi.org/10.1017/S1092852919001366.
4. Reddon H, Gueant JL, Meyre D. The importance of gene-environment interactions in human obesity. Clin Sci (Lond). 2016;130(18):1571–97. https://doi.org/10.1042/cs20160221.
5. Bray GA, Kim KK, Wilding JPH. Obesity: a chronic relapsing progressive disease process. A position statement of the World Obesity Federation. Obes Rev. 2017;18(7):715–23. https://doi.org/10.1111/obr.12551.
6. Wharton S, Lau DCW, Vallis M, Sharma AM, Biertho L, Campbell-Scherer D, et al. Obesity in adults: a clinical practice guideline. CMAJ. 2020;192(31):E875–E91. https://doi.org/10.1503/cmaj.191707.
7. Dalle Grave R, Calugi S. Cognitive behavior therapy for adolescents with eating disorders. New York: Guilford Press; 2020.
8. Schmidt R, Tetzlaff A, Hilbert A. Perceived expressed emotion in adolescents with binge-eating disorder. J Abnorm Child Psychol. 2015;43(7):1369–77. https://doi.org/10.1007/s10802-015-0015-x.
9. van Furth EF, van Strien DC, Martina LM, van Son MJ, Hendrickx JJ, van Engeland H. Expressed emotion and the prediction of outcome in adolescent eating disorders. Int J Eat Disord. 1996;20(1):19–31. https://doi.org/10.1002/(sici)1098-108x(199607)20:1<19::Aid-eat3>3.0.Co;2-7.

Review Session: Taking Stock 11

Abstract

A review session is scheduled for the end of Step One to review the treatment progress and to plan for Step Two. Progress should be reviewed jointly, and any emerging obstacles to change identified. The personal formulation should be reviewed and updated if necessary, and the next stage of the treatment planned, selecting specific modules to address the psychopathology operating in the individual patient, as appropriate. The Healthy Weight Loss module is recommended when a patient with clinical or non-clinical obesity has significantly reduced their binge-eating episodes and does not display overvaluation of shape and weight or a personal history of anorexia nervosa or bulimia nervosa. A subgroup of patients with binge-eating disorder (BED) achieves a complete remission of binge-eating episodes, has no other signs of eating-disorder psychopathology, and does not aim to lose weight after the end of Step One. In such cases, the treatment continues with the procedures described in the Setbacks and Mindsets and Maintenance Preparation modules.

11.1 Structure and Content

The progression of CBT for BED is collaboratively assessed with the patient every week through the collaborative measurement and interpretation of weight and analysis of the EPCL-BED (see Table A2 and Appendix 3). In addition to the weekly assessment, at the end of Step One a portion of the session is dedicated to reviewing the treatment progress and planning for Step Two. The review has the following objectives:

- To conduct a joint review of progress
- To identify any emerging obstacles to change

R. Dalle Grave et al., *Cognitive Behavior Therapy for Binge Eating Disorder*, https://doi.org/10.1007/978-3-031-71456-6_11

- To review and, if necessary, update the personal formulation
- To design and plan the rest of the treatment

Simultaneously, the procedures introduced in Step One continue to be implemented. In this phase of the treatment, the session frequency changes from twice to once a week.

11.2 Conducting a Joint Review of Progresses

Studies on CBT for eating disorders have found that the extent of improvements achieved in the first four weeks of treatment, particularly a reduction in the frequency of binge-eating episodes, predicts treatment outcome [1]. For this reason, the patient is encouraged to "start well" and strive for maximum behavioural change during Step One.

Treatment trial results also suggest that if progress is limited, it is crucial to quickly recognize and understand the reasons why and implement potential solutions. Therefore, a formal and detailed review of the patient's progress should be conducted at this point in the programme. If progress is limited, it should be promptly acknowledged, and the treatment modified to overcome the identified obstacles to change.

At this stage it is also helpful to ask the patient to complete the self-administered questionnaires EDE-Q [2, 3] and CIA [4, 5], which they already filled out at the beginning of treatment, to get an objective assessment of the nature and extent of the changes made thus far. Indeed, patients with BED often tend to underestimate their progress, and therefore need assistance in considering all their improvements in a balanced manner. In cases in which the programme is progressing well, the patient typically reports a reduction in both weight concern and the frequency of binge-eating episodes after 4 weeks (due to the collaborative weighing and regular eating procedures, respectively), while in most cases concerns about body shape usually do not change because they have not yet been addressed by the treatment.

It is also a good idea at this point to discuss with the patient which aspects of the treatment, in their opinion, have helped them make progress, to reinforce the therapeutic procedures already being implemented. The therapist should always praise the patient and attribute the change to their efforts.

11.3 Identifying Any Obstacles

The second goal of the review session is to identify any obstacles to change. This involves assessing the patient's attitudes toward treatment and using procedures outlined in CBT for BED. The assessment should be done openly, introducing the topic to the patient in this way: "*I think this is the right time to review not only the progress you have made but also your attitude towards treatment. Are you satisfied with how things are going? Do you think the treatment is suitable for your problem? Is there anything you would like to discuss?*" Then, after hearing the patient's point of view, the therapist might say to the patient: "*Now, I would like to examine with you to what extent you have been able to use the treatment procedures to help you change. I have a table listing the various elements of the treatment introduced so far. Would you mind if we analyse them together?*" Then, the therapist and patient discuss the elements described in Table 11.1.

If problems are identified in the engagement or use of specific treatment procedures, the therapist should explore their origin. Generally, these issues arise from the eating-disorder psychopathology and/or more general factors. In some cases, the processes maintaining the eating disorder are so powerful and ingrained that they prevent the patient from making agreed-upon changes, despite their best efforts to do so. For example, some patients continue to experience binge-eating episodes even with the adoption of the regular eating procedure. Typically, in patients with BED, this is because their eating is strongly influenced by events and emotions and, in a minority of cases, they still adhere to dysfunctional eating patterns that have not yet been addressed in treatment. In other cases, a patient may continue to weigh themselves at home out of fear of gaining weight, or due to the desire to lose weight. A review of such obstacles should be done with reference to the patient's personal formulation. The main obstacles that generally hinder improvement are the following:

- *Clinical depression.* As described in Chap. 4, clinical depression often coexists with BED and, if present, negatively interacts with the eating disorder and the patient's ability to benefit from the programme. Those with clinical depression may believe that change is not possible, lack the energy to engage in treatment, and have insufficient concentration to understand and retain information. In such cases, treating clinical depression with antidepressant medication is imperative. Sect. 4.8.1 describes how to distinguish coexisting clinical depression from that secondary to the eating disorder, and how to treat it.
- *Interpersonal difficulties.* People with BED and higher weight often report interpersonal difficulties of various kinds that contribute to maintaining the eating disorder and hinder treatment. Two examples are (1) "interpersonal instability",

Table 11.1 Treatment elements review

	How the treatment is going		
Treatment elements	Not well	Well enough	Well
Attending sessions			
Being on time			
Not weighing at home			
Monitoring in real time			
Regular eating			
Addressing sedentary lifestyle			
Making the treatment a priority			
Playing an active role in treatment			
Others			

which derails treatment or reduces adherence to tasks between sessions; and (2) "interpersonal void", an absence of meaningful relationships, which the patient may be using binge eating to mitigate. In such cases, the proactive problem-solving procedure should be implemented (see Chap. 13).

- *Mood intolerance.* In a subgroup of individuals with BED, eating is markedly influenced by events and associated mood changes. These individuals suffer from a problem called "mood intolerance," which contributes to maintaining binge-eating episodes and hinders treatment. In such cases, the procedures described in Chap. 13 should be applied.
- *Competing commitments.* Work or other commitments may not allow the patient to dedicate enough time to the programme. In such cases, we emphasize that the treatment will only work if it is given priority. To find a workable solution to this problem, the pros and cons of temporarily setting aside other commitments to give priority to their recovery should be collaboratively assessed with the patient.
- *Difficulty adapting to CBT.* Some patients, particularly those who have undergone long courses of psychotherapy aimed at analyzing the hypothetical causes of their eating disorder, may find it difficult to adapt to a programme mainly focused on overcoming maintenance mechanisms. If this seems to be the patient's main obstacle to progress, we invite them to put aside any scepticism and try to rigorously apply the strategies and procedures of the programme, whose effects have been extensively evaluated by research. A minority of patients report wanting a treatment that results in "rapid" weight loss. In such cases, we review with the patient whether previous attempts at rapid weight loss have been successful. In any event, we encourage them to stick with our programme, which has the ambitious objective of their overcoming the eating disorder and, at the same time, gradually reaching a healthy weight.

11.4 Reviewing the Personal Formulation

The review conducted after 4 weeks is an opportunity to perform a formal and detailed reassessment of the initial personal formulation. For this purpose, the therapist should review the patient's monitoring records with them, jointly assessing whether any maintenance processes have emerged that need to be added to the formulation, and whether others may no longer seem relevant in maintaining the eating-disorder psychopathology and therefore need to be crossed off. If significant changes are noted, redrawing the personalized formulation on a new sheet of paper may be helpful.

11.5 Planning Step Two

During Step Two, the procedures introduced in Step One continue to be applied, and one or more of the following maintenance processes are addressed via specific modules:

- *Overvaluation of shape and weight.* This form of psychopathology has been found in about 50% of patients with BED [6]. If present, it should be addressed at the beginning of Step Two via the Body Image module, as individuals who adopt dysfunctional dietary restriction attempts may be having difficulty reducing their binge-eating episodes. Typical expressions of the overvaluation of shape and excessive weight to be addressed include marginalizing other areas of life, and body checking and avoidance.
- *Clinical or non-clinical obesity.* The Healthy Weight Loss module is indicated for patients who have clinical obesity (see Sect. 4.3.1 and Table 4.4 for the definition) and significantly reduced binge-eating episodes and do not show signs of the overvaluation of shape and weight or a personal history of anorexia nervosa or bulimia nervosa. Although primarily intended for patients who have clinical obesity, the module is also suitable for those with non-clinical obesity who desire to achieve moderate, healthy weight loss. In such patients, the aim is to replace dysregulated eating and overeating with a healthy eating pattern, with a view to preventing the onset of clinical obesity or other non-communicable diseases.
- *Unhealthy and rigid dietary restraint.* In Step Two, the regular eating procedure initiated in Step One is continued. At the same time, strict dietary restriction is addressed through the strategies and procedures of the Dysfunctional Dieting module.
- *Events and mood changes.* Events and associated mood changes often trigger a modification in eating behaviour (e.g., binge-eating episodes, dysregulated eating and/or overeating) in patients with BED [7]. If residual binge episodes persist and are associated with events and mood changes, the Events, Moods and Eating module should be implemented in Step Two.
- *Unrealistic weight-loss and primary goals.* The Unrealistic Goals module is indicated for patients who are working through the Healthy Weight Loss module but have high weight-loss expectations and other primary goals (e.g., improving interpersonal relationships and/or self-confidence, finding a partner or a new job) that they link to these expectations [8], as these are associated with a higher dropout rate [9, 10] and with the adoption of dysfunctional dieting that in turn contributes to the maintenance of binge-eating episodes. The aim is to help the patient be satisfied with a reasonable and healthy weight loss by striking a balance between what can be changed and what must be accepted.
- *Internalized weight stigma.* The Internalized Weight Stigma module is indicated for patients with internalized weight stigma, as this is associated with negative emotions that often trigger episodes of binge eating and overeating (Fig. 2.1) [11]. At the same time, the low self-efficacy associated with internalized weight stigma [12] can lead to failing in or excessive devotion to the attempt to control eating end weight.
- *Setbacks and maintenance preparation.* Toward the end of Step Two, the Setbacks and Mindsets and Maintenance Preparation modules are introduced in preparation for further work on staying well in the future, which will be the focus of Step Three of treatment.

Generally speaking, Step Two is begun with the Healthy Weight Loss and Dysfunctional Dieting modules for patients in whom it is medically advisable. Then, the strategies and procedures of the Events, Moods, and Eating module can be introduced if the patient is experiencing residual binge-eating episodes associated with events and mood changes. Finally, unrealistic weight-loss goals other primary goals are addressed in the later stages of Step Two if a decrease in satisfaction with lost weight is observed. However, if the patient presents the overvaluation of shape and weight, weight loss is not indicated. Instead, it is advisable to start Step Two by addressing body image, because this is one of the most potent maintenance mechanisms and takes a long time to overcome. After 1 or 2 weeks, the strategies and procedures suggested in the Events, Moods and Eating module can be introduced. The sequence can be reversed if events and emotions are deemed predominant in maintaining the disorder. It is reccomended to address internalized weight stigma in the early phase of Step Two in all the patients reporting these psychological poblem.

A subgroup of patients with BED achieves complete remission from binge-eating episodes, does not report other eating-disorder psychopathology, and does not aim to lose weight after the end of Step One. In such cases, the treatment should continue with the procedures described in the Setbacks and Mindsets and Maintenance Preparation modules. In any event, it is advisable to be flexible and adapt the strategies and procedures based on changes in the individual's eating disorder and weight. The patient should be continuously encouraged to make the treatment a priority and help maintain the momentum for change introduced in Step One.

Vignette

The patient, a 27-year-old woman with a BMI of 31, has been suffering from BED since the age of 25. After the end of a 5-year romantic relationship, binge-eating episodes without compensatory behaviours began, leading to a weight gain of approximately 20 kg over the course of 2 years. The patient unsuccessfully underwent psychoanalysis-oriented psychotherapy for about a year, and then attempted, without success, to follow a ketogenic diet prescribed by a nutritionist. The patient began CBT for BED enthusiastically, appreciating the collaborative nature of the treatment, which aims to address binge-eating episodes but not weight loss initially. During Step One, she diligently implemented the agreed-upon procedures, significantly reducing the frequency of binge-eating episodes (from about two per day to two per week). However, despite adopting the regular eating procedure, she continued to maintain extreme and rigid dietary rules (no carbohydrate intake except for during binge-eating episodes), motivated by the desire to return to her weight before the onset of BED. During the review session, it became clear that residual binge-eating episodes, during which she consumed large quantities of carbohydrate-rich foods, were primarily maintained by adopting extreme and rigid dietary rules, prompted by the overvaluation of shape and weight. The patient reported that shape and weight had become the most important domain in her self-evaluation scheme. Furthermore, she avoided exposing her body by wearing loose, black clothes, and engaged in numerous dysfunctional body-checking behaviours in front of a mirror at home, reinforcing her disdain for her body. After collaboratively reviewing the mechanisms maintaining her residual binge-eating episodes and redrawing her personalized formulation, the patient agreed to address the overvaluation of shape and weight and dysfunctional dietary restraint in Step Two and not to focus on weight loss.

References

1. Fairburn CG, Agras WS, Walsh BT, Wilson GT, Stice E. Prediction of outcome in bulimia nervosa by early change in treatment. Am J Psychiatry. 2004;161(12):2322–4.
2. Calugi S, Milanese C, Sartirana M, El Ghoch M, Sartori F, Geccherle E, et al. The eating disorder examination questionnaire: reliability and validity of the Italian version. Eat Weight Disord. 2017;22(3):509–14. https://doi.org/10.1007/s40519-016-0276-6.
3. Fairburn CG, Cooper Z, O'Connor M. Eating Disorder Examination Questionnaire (EDE-Q 6.0). In: Fairburn CG, editor. Cognitive behavior therapy and eating disorders. New York: Guilford Press; 2008. p. 309–13.
4. Calugi S, Sartirana M, Milanese C, El Ghoch M, Riolfi F, Dalle GR. The clinical impairment assessment questionnaire: validation in Italian patients with eating disorders. Eat Weight Disord. 2018;23(5):685–94. https://doi.org/10.1007/s40519-018-0477-2.
5. Bohn K, Doll HA, Cooper Z, O'Connor M, Palmer RL, Fairburn CG. The measurement of impairment due to eating disorder psychopathology. Behav Res Ther. 2008;46(10):1105–10. https://doi.org/10.1016/j.brat.2008.06.012.
6. Grilo CM, Hrabosky JI, White MA, Allison KC, Stunkard AJ, Masheb RM. Overvaluation of shape and weight in binge eating disorder and overweight controls: refinement of a diagnostic construct. J Abnorm Psychol. 2008;117(2):414–9. https://doi.org/10.1037/0021-843x.117.2.414.
7. Nicholls W, Devonport TJ, Blake M. The association between emotions and eating behaviour in an obese population with binge eating disorder. Obes Rev. 2016;17(1):30–42. https://doi.org/10.1111/obr.12329.
8. Dalle Grave R, Calugi S, Magri F, Cuzzolaro M, Dall'aglio E, Lucchin L, et al. Weight loss expectations in obese patients seeking treatment at medical centers. Obes Res. 2004;12(12):2005–12. https://doi.org/10.1038/oby.2004.251.
9. Calugi S, Marchesini G, El Ghoch M, Gavasso I, Dalle GR. The association between weight maintenance and session-by-session diet adherence, weight loss and weight-loss satisfaction. Eat Weight Disord. 2020;25(1):127–33. https://doi.org/10.1007/s40519-018-0528-8.
10. Dalle Grave R, Calugi S, Molinari E, Petroni ML, Bondi M, Compare A, et al. Weight loss expectations in obese patients and treatment attrition: an observational multicenter study. Obes Res. 2005;13(11):1961–9. https://doi.org/10.1038/oby.2005.241.
11. Calugi S, Segattini B, Cattaneo G, Chimini M, Dalle Grave A, Dametti L, et al. Weight bias internalization and eating disorder psychopathology in treatment-seeking patients with obesity. Nutrients. 2023;15(13) https://doi.org/10.3390/nu15132932.
12. Himmelstein MS, Puhl RM, Pearl RL, Pinto AM, Foster GD. Coping with weight stigma among adults in a commercial weight management sample. Int J Behav Med 2020;27(5):576–90. https://doi.org/10.1007/s12529-020-09895-4.

Healthy Weight Loss Module 12

Abstract

This module is intended for patients with clinical obesity who are motivated to achieve reasonable and healthy weight loss, and for those with non-clinical obesity who want to improve their overall health and prevent the development of clinical obesity and other non-communicable diseases. The module is not indicated for patients who have not adopted a regular eating pattern and reduced the frequency of binge-eating episodes, or for those with the overvaluation of shape and weight or a history of anorexia nervosa or bulimia nervosa. The module aims to help the patient (i) achieve, accept, and maintain a reasonable and healthy weight loss; (ii) adopt a lifestyle that promotes long-term weight control; and (iii) develop a stable, healthy weight-control mindset. To achieve these goals, the patient is helped to adopt moderate and flexible dietary restriction, as opposed to extreme and rigid dietary restriction, based on healthy eating guidelines. This is associated with the remission of binge-eating episodes and can help the patient achieve a reasonable and healthy weight loss (i.e., a 5–10%). In patients with indications to lose weight that have difficulties adhering to moderate and flexible dietary restriction, the new weight incretin-based weight-loss drugs can be considered.

Recent research seems to indicate that dietary restraint is not a singular entity. There is preliminary evidence indicating that flexible dietary restraint, as opposed to rigid restraint, does not impede binge-eating control in people with BED, instead being linked to both the cessation of binge eating and improved weight loss [1, 2]. Hence, this module is indicated for patients with BED and clinical obesity such as to cause alterations in the function of tissues, organs or the individual due to excessive and/or abnormal adiposity (e.g., arterial hypertension, type 2 diabetes, obstructive sleep apnoea syndrome, non-alcoholic fatty liver disease, arthritis, physical functional impairments, see also Sect. 4.3.1 and Table 4.4 for the definition). There should, however, be strong evidence that these obesity-related complications would be improved by a reasonable amount of weight loss, and the patient does need to be motivated to achieve it [3].

R. Dalle Grave et al., *Cognitive Behavior Therapy for Binge Eating Disorder*,
https://doi.org/10.1007/978-3-031-71456-6_12

The module may also be suitable for people with non-clinical obesity who wish to improve their overall health and prevent the onset of clinical obesity and other non-communicable diseases, but not necessarily reduce weight-related harm [4]. That being said, we always discuss with such patients that treatment of non-clinical obesity does not necessarily have to focus on weight loss, as adopting a healthy lifestyle might be a better goal than weight loss in preventing cardiovascular and general mortality [5–7]. The module is not indicated for patients with overvaluation of shape and weight, a history of anorexia nervosa or bulimia nervosa, and in those with major depression or other not stable severe mental disorders.

The Healthy Weight Loss module is introduced if the patient meets the above criteria and has successfully adopted a regular eating pattern and markedly reduced the frequency of binge-eating episodes during Step One of CBT for BED. At the same time strategies to deal with residual binge-eating episodes are implemented. The weight-loss phase should last approximately 24 weeks, and be followed by an indefinite period of weight maintenance (see Step 3).

12.1 The Main Goals of the Module

12.1.1 Achieving, Accepting, and Maintaining Reasonable and Healthy Weight Loss

Several studies have shown that it is not necessary for people with clinical obesity to lose a large amount of weight to reduce the impact of weight-related medical complications. In most cases, a modest weight loss is sufficient. For instance, a 5–10% reduction in body weight has been observed to improve health-related quality of life significantly (HRQoL) [8], as well as reducing cardiovascular risk factors [9], the risk of developing type 2 diabetes in predisposed individuals [10], and most other medical complications associated with clinical obesity [9, 11, 12]. One study demonstrated that a 15% weight loss leads to remission of type 2 diabetes in patients with diabetes lasting less than 6 years [13]. Recently, another study has found that a $\geq$ 5 to <10% weight loss in patients with BED is associated with significant improvements in HDL, triglycerides, HbA1c, and mean plasma glucose, whereas $\geq$10% weight loss is associated with significant improvements in all cardiovascular disease risk factors (except blood pressure) at 12-month follow-up [14]. Research carried out by our team has shown that moderate weight loss achieved by patients with clinical obesity who underwent CBT is also correlated with a significant improvement in body image [15], depression, and anxiety [16].

From these studies, the concept of "reasonable and healthy weight loss" has emerged, which can be defined as "the weight loss that can be achieved by adopting a flexible, moderately calorie-restricted healthy diet and an active lifestyle". In most cases, this corresponds to a weight loss ranging from 5% to 10% [17] (see Table 12.1), which is associated with a significant improvements in complications associated with clinical obesity. There is also good evidence that such improvements are maintained if the weight is not regained.

Table 12.1 Percentage of weight loss associated with significant clinical improvements in major complications associated with clinical obesity

Arterial hypertension ≥5%
Hypercholesterolemia ≥5%
Hypertriglyceridemia ≥5%
Type 2 diabetes prevention ≥5%
Type 2 diabetes remission[a] ≥15%
Incidence of cardiovascular diseases ≥10%
Metabolic dysfunction-associated fatty liver disease (MAFLD) ≥5%
Metabolic dysfunction-associated steatohepatitis (MASH) ≥10–40%
Osteoarthritis >10%, ≥5% if associated with excessive physical exercise
Asthma ≥7–8%
Obstructive sleep apnoea ≥7–11%
PCOS, fertility issues, hirsutism ≥10%
Low testosterone levels ≥5–15%
Stress incontinence ≥5–10%
Gastroesophageal reflux disease (GERD) ≥10%
HRQoL ≥5%

[a]Of less than 6 years duration

12.1.2 Adopting a Healthy Lifestyle

The goal of making reasonable and healthy weight control a central part of life distinguishes this programme from traditional dietary treatments. This distinction can be broken down into three fundamental points:

1. CBT for BED emphasizes that losing and maintaining weight requires a long-term change (for life) because clinical obesity is a chronic condition.
2. It shifts the emphasis from physical appearance (a motivating factor commonly associated with treatment interruption) to physical health. Individuals are taught the importance of developing a healthy lifestyle to achieve significant health benefits, regardless of the total weight lost.
3. It directs the patient's attention away from the unpredictable nature of weight modification in favour of more controllable lifestyle changes.

12.1.3 Developing a Healthy, Stable, and Flexible Weight-Control Mindset

Similarly, the goal of a "healthy weight-control mindset" distinguishes this treatment from traditional weight-loss programmes that pay little attention to cognitive processes influencing weight control, as their main purpose is to change eating behaviour and physical activity levels.

12.2 Adopting Moderate and Flexible Dietary Restriction

The key to managing BED and higher weight is to adhere to a healthy diet based on flexible dietary guidelines and include a reasonable combination of foods, including enjoyable ones. We suggest that the patient adopt a dietary plan involving moderate caloric restriction (approximately 500 kcal per day) to achieve a variable weight loss of about 0.5 kg per week. We provide the patient with a flexible dietary plan based on the Italian Mediterranean diet, tailored to their personal preferences, characteristics and metabolic goals. The choice to adopt this dietary model stems from its proven long-term effectiveness in weight loss, as compared to a low-fat diet [18]. Furthermore, the Mediterranean diet is known for its health benefits [5, 19], and is preferred by the population we treat. However, the dietary plan can be easily adapted to different cultures, patient preferences, and health conditions, as suggested by AHA/ACC/TOS guidelines, by employing one of the following methods to reduce food and calorie intake [9]:

- Subtracting 500 kcal from the patient's daily intake if weight has remained stable over the last 4 weeks.
- Suggesting a dietary plan comprising 1200–1500 kcal/day for women and 1500–1800 kcal/day for men (kcal levels should be adjusted based on individual weight).
- Recommending any evidence-based dietary plan that limits specific types of foods (such as high-carbohydrate, low-fibre foods, or high-fat foods) to create an energy deficit through moderate and flexible dietary restriction.

Moderate and flexible dietary restriction does not increase the risk of binge-eating episodes, and can help the patient achieve a healthy weight loss (e.g., $\geq 5\%$ of baseline weight) [9]. There is also evidence that moderate and flexible dietary restriction, as opposed to extreme and rigid dietary restriction, is associated with remission of binge-eating episodes [1, 2].

12.2.1 Planning When, What, and Where to Eat

We explain to patients that planning *what* to eat and drink increases adherence to moderate dietary restriction, and is crucial for changing eating habits that are automatic and seemingly difficult to modify [20]. We remind them that they have already experienced the effectiveness of planning when making changes to their meal schedule, and suggest to them that now is the time to focus on what and how much to eat, now that they have adopted the regular eating procedure.

To assist the patient in improving the quality of their diet, we provide meal plans based on exchanging options within food groups, as published by the American Diabetes Association and the American Dietetic Association [21] and adapted for the Italian Mediterranean diet [20]. The system is designed to create a caloric deficit of about 500 kcal per day relative to the estimated total energy expenditure [22].[1] In our clinical practice, the mean plan is explained over the course of a couple of sessions with an in-house dietician, who has had specific training on the nature and style of CBT for BED.

The main advantage of the food exchange system is that it provides the patient with a wide selection of foods, offering variety and versatility to individuals trying to limit their calorie intake. Additionally, by grouping foods with similar nutritional content, it can help patients make flexible substitutions based on their preferences without exceeding their calorie goal. However, the patient is informed that the "menus" we provide should be taken as a general guide that they should use to create a personalized and flexible meal plan based on their individual preferences and lifestyle. It is not realistic to expect adherence to a prescribed meal plan indefinitely, and the goal of CBT for BED is for the patient to gradually learn to manage their own eating and weight issues. From our clinical experience, we have observed that patients who are taught to count calories but told that the aim is to adhere to an approximate, not strict, daily intake become more aware of the calorie content of foods and their impact on energy balance. This awareness helps them choose foods with lower energy density, become more flexible in meal planning, and better adhere to a moderate and flexible dietary restriction that makes binge-eating episodes less likely.

We also discuss with the patient how to reduce their portion sizes, as downsizing meals is a crucial strategy for weight control [23]. We also provide them with the following general guidelines:

- Weigh food before cooking (if possible).
- Use easy-to-follow reference measurements to estimate food portions (e.g., a cup for 80 g of rice, a glass for a serving of milk, a spoon for 10 g of olive oil).
- Consume only pre-packaged foods with indicated calorie content.
- Choose restaurants that serve normal-sized portions (i.e., smaller portions).
- Use smaller plates (a strategy that helps reduce portion sizes).
- Food should be served only once and in the right portion (no second helpings).

In the initial weeks of making such changes to their eating habits, we suggest that the patient limit social occasions on which they might be exposed to numerous food stimuli and find it difficult to plan what to eat. Indeed, one of the primary early goals of the treatment is to help the patient adopt new eating habits, interrupting dysregulated eating and overeating, which is easier to do when they eat in an environment in which temptation is reduced and they have complete control over what to eat. Hence, the patient should ideally plan to consume as many meals as possible at home or in restaurants where they know the menu and the calorie composition of the

[1] In obesity treatment trials, total energy expenditure is usually estimated by multiplying the Basal Metabolic Rate (BMR), which can be estimated via FAO/WHO/UNU equations [22], by a Physical Activity Level (PAL) value of 1.3. For example, a female with a PAL of 1.3 and a mean BMR of 1500 kcal/day would have a mean energy requirement of $1.3 \times 1600 = 1950$ kcal/day).

Table 12.2 Information provided to patients for planning moderate and flexible dietary restriction

Planning ahead when, what, and where to eat and eating consciously helps you stick to moderate, flexible dietary restriction. It will also help you to adopt a meal plan that aligns with your preferences rather than force yourself to eat things you do not enjoy.
When to eat:
Adopt a regular eating schedule (have planned snacks between main meals and avoid consuming anything between).
What to eat:
A healthy weight loss of approximately 0.5 kg/week can be achieved by creating an energy deficit of 500 kcal/day. As weight loss progresses, it is necessary to slightly reduce calorie content to achieve the same weekly weight loss due to a decrease in resting energy expenditure.
Two main strategies exist to achieve this energy deficit: (i) follow a diet that limits certain types of foods (e.g., high-carbohydrate, low-fibre, or high-fat foods) or (ii) counting calories.
However, research tells us that weight loss does not depend on the composition of the diet but on calorie control [24].
We therefore suggest calorie-counting and a meal plan based on the Mediterranean diet.
The Mediterranean diet reduces the risk of cardiovascular diseases [5] and related risk factors such as waist-to-hip ratio, lipid levels, and inflammation markers. It also lessens the risk of developing breast cancer, depression, colorectal cancer, diabetes, obesity, asthma, erectile dysfunction, and cognitive decline [25].
The Mediterranean diet aligns with healthy eating guidelines derived from the Harvard University (USA) association between nutrition and disease development, as indicated by the Harvard healthy eating plate https://www.hsph.harvard.edu/nutritionsource/healthy-eating-plate/
Where to eat:
In the early weeks, limit social occasions with significant exposure to food stimuli.
Plan to eat most meals at home or in restaurants where the menu and calorie composition of dishes is known.
After developing new eating habits, work on handling social occasions. Continue real-time self-monitoring of food intake.

dishes served (enabling advance meal planning). During meals at home, we encourage patients to eat only at the kitchen or dining table. Once the patient has developed new eating habits and feels in control of their diet, they are encouraged not to avoid scheduled social occasions and, subsequently, to accept sudden invitations to lunch or dinner. These will be the perfect opportunities to test their ability to control their eating without being influenced by the external environment.

Table 12.2 summarizes the essential information we give patients to help them plan moderate and flexible dietary restriction.

12.3 Continuing Real-Time Self-Monitoring

We encourage patients to persist with real-time self-monitoring using the methods learned in previous weeks, as this strategy helps change some automatic eating habits and enhances adherence to meal planning [26]. We instruct patients to briefly describe the events, thoughts and emotions associated with any deviation from the meal plan in the Comments column.

Figure 12.1 provides an example of a monitoring record showing both the meal plan ("Today's Plan") and the real-time monitoring carried out by a patient. Note that the column "kcal" has been added to the monitoring record introduced in Step One of the treatment.

12.4 Eating Consciously

Another key strategy that can help improve adherence to moderate and flexible caloric restriction and interrupt dysfunctional automatic eating habits is conscious eating. This involves the patient *observing their behaviour* during meals. For this reason, we suggest the patient eat slowly, savour each bite, appreciate the smell,

Day *15th March* **Date** *Monday*

Time	Food and drink consumed	Place	*	Calories	Comments
7 am	*Plan for Today*				
	1 glass of semi-skim milk	*Kitchen*		*75*	
	3 whole wheat toast			*10*	
10:30 am	*1 orange*	*Work*		*75*	
1 pm	*1 plate of pasta (80 g)*	*Work*		*300*	
	Tomato sauce 50 g			*10*	
	Parmesan cheese 1			*40*	
	tablespoon			*40*	
	Mixed salad 200 g			*90*	
	Olive oil 1 tablespoon			*90*	
	1 golden apple			*60*	
4:30 pm	*1 fruit yogurt (125 g)*	*Work*		*250*	
8 pm	*Chicken breast 200 g*	*Kitchen*		*40*	
	Mixed salad 200 g			*90*	
	Olive oil 1 tablespoon			*90*	
	5 whole wheat crackers			*90*	
	1 golden apple			*1350*	
7 am	*1 glass of semi-skim milk*	*Kitchen*		*75*	
	3 whole wheat toast			*10*	
10:30 am	*1 orange*	*Work*		*75*	
1 pm	*1 plate of pasta (80 g)*	*Work*		*300*	
	Tomato sauce 50 g			*10*	
	Parmesan cheese 1			*40*	
	tablespoon			*40*	
	Mixed salad 200 g			*90*	
	Olive oil 1 tablespoon			*90*	
	1 golden apple			*220*	
4:30 pm	*1 ice cream*	*Bar*	*	*250*	*I was craving something sweet, and I saw my colleague eating an ice cream*
8 pm	*Chicken breast 200 g*	*Kitchen*		*40*	
	Mixed salad 200 g			*90*	
	Olive oil 1 tablespoon			*90*	
	5 whole wheat crackers			*90*	
	1 golden apple			*1510*	*The day went well anyway, I didn't binge and ate regularly.*
Steps		Number: *8,000*			
Formal exercise		Type:			Minutes:

Fig. 12.1 Example of a monitoring record filled in by a patient for meal planning and self-monitoring in real time

texture, colour, and taste of food, and adopt a mindset focused on weight control. Conscious eating also involves following the meal plan without being influenced by external factors (e.g., the sight of food, life events) or internal stimuli (e.g., food cravings, need for gratification, hunger, thoughts about food, mood changes). This cognitive approach to eating, facilitated by real-time food monitoring, should be adopted by the patient until they develop new healthy eating habits and can trust their internal hunger and fullness cues to regulate eating more naturally. We also inform the patient that to achieve this state, they will need to practice conscious eating for several weeks until they realize they have developed new eating habits that do not require much cognitive effort to maintain.

We also encourage patients to adopt a goal-oriented mindset, geared towards the long-term objectives of treatment (e.g., achieving healthy weight loss and related physical and psychological benefits). This cognitive strategy can help them tolerate short-term adverse experiences (e.g., hunger and cravings for highly palatable foods) that may occur when reducing energy intake.

12.4.1 Addressing Patient Questions and Concerns

The therapist should always inquire whether the patient has any doubts or questions about meal planning procedures, real-time self-monitoring and eating consciously. Here are a few examples of typical concerns and appropriate responses:

Patient: Can I follow the menu without counting calories?

Therapist: Yes, you could. However, I suggest counting calories for a while because it will make you more aware of the energy content of what you eat, and this will help you create a personalized and flexible meal plan based on your preferences and lifestyle.

Patient: Eating consciously all the time is so complicated!

Therapist: Yes, it is challenging and somewhat unnatural. However, it's a procedure you should apply for several weeks to improve your control over eating. If you eat consciously, you'll be better able to handle impulses to deviate from your meal plan and decide what to eat or not eat. Once you've developed new eating habits that don't require a lot of thought, you'll be able to eat more naturally.

12.5 If and When to Prescribe Weight-Loss Drugs

The new incretin-based medications are a class of antidiabetic drugs that stabilize blood glucose by stimulating insulin secretion and suppressing glucagon production in the body in response to energy intake [27]. In addition to their hypoglycaemic effects, some of these drugs (i.e., liraglutide, semaglutide, and tirzepatide) have been shown to be highly effective in facilitating weight control through lifestyle changes [28], and have been approved by the Food and Drug Administration (FDA) for the chronic management of obesity.

In people with obesity or overweight and weight-related comorbidities (but not diabetes), 3 mg liraglutide, a glucagon-like peptide-1 receptor agonist (GLP-1RA), reduced baseline body weight by 8% by 56 weeks [29], while 2.4 mg semaglutide, another GLP-1RA, produced a weight loss of 15% over 2 years [30]. Both drugs decrease energy intake mainly by modifying hunger and satiety signals in specific neural regions and slowing gastric emptying [31]. Tirzepatide, a dual agonist for glucose-dependent insulinotropic polypeptide (GIP) and GLP-1 RAs, has synergistic effects on appetite, energy intake, and fat mass [32]. 15 mg produced an average weight loss of 20.9% after 72 weeks [33].

Semaglutide 2.4 has also been shown to produce a 20% reduction in the risk of heart attack or stroke in non-diabetic patients with overweight or obesity and established cardiovascular disease [34]. Furthermore, it has been shown to improve symptoms, physical limitations, and exercise function, and reduce inflammation and body weight in patients with obesity and heart failure with preserved ejection fraction [35]. Tirzepatide has demonstrated similar positive effects in individuals with clinical obesity and also a clinical improvement of obstructive sleep apnoea [36].

Despite these important positive clinical effects, some problems are associated with the use of the new weight-loss drugs. Here are the main ones:

1. *Side effects*. Common side effects include nausea, abdominal pain, vomiting, diarrhoea, and constipation [37]. These side effects sometimes get better over time. They can be prevented and moderated by titrating the drug's dose upward over 16 to 20 weeks, eating slowly and in small portions, stopping eating when one is full, not skipping meals, and avoiding fatty, fried, and greasy foods. However, at least 10% of patients who start these drugs have to be taken off them because the side effects do not improve. It should also be underlined that GLP-1RAs can be associated with rare but more severe side effects (e.g., pancreatitis, hypoglycaemia, diabetic retinopathy complications, gastroparesis, and bowel obstruction) [37, 38]. Research on the long-term use of GLP-1ARs is ongoing, and additional side effects may continue to emerge [39].
2. *Excessive loss of lean body mass (LBM)*. Weight loss with semaglutide and tirzepatide results in beneficial reductions in body fat but also decreases lean body mass (LBM). This reduction in LBM can lower daily energy expenditure, impacting long-term weight maintenance, and is associated with decreased bone mineral density and increased fracture risk [40]. Adults over 65 are particularly at risk for sarcopenia, an age-related loss of muscle mass, strength, and function [41]. Intensive lifestyle interventions typically result in 15–25% of weight loss from LBM [42], but with semaglutide, this can reach the 40% [43]. Some LBM loss is expected during weight loss, especially from low-density muscle, which may reduce concerns. Prioritizing large-scale studies on body composition changes with these medications is crucial to identify risk factors for excessive lean mass loss, including age, gender, and weight loss rate.
3. *High rate of discontinuation*. A discontinuation of the GLP-1RAs greater than 50% in patiens with obesity has been reported A discontinuation rate of greater than 50% for GLP-1RAs in patients with obesity has been reported [44]. Several

factors may lead patients to discontinuing these drugs including [40] concerns about their long-term safety; patients' beliefs that they should now be able to control their weight on their own; and the continued high costs of AOMs for weight-loss maintenance. Indeed, the drugs are costly (up to $1300/month in the US and €300/month in Europe), and not usually provided by national health systems or covered by health insurance providers. The use of these drugs is, therefore, prohibitive for many people with clinical obesity.

4. *Weight regain.* With semaglutide, weight loss reaches a plateau after 62 weeks, and two-thirds of the weight is regained if the drug is discontinued [45]. A similar rate of weight regain has also been observed after the discontinuation of tirzepatide [46]. These findings indicate that they should be used as "lifetime drugs" in the management of clinical obesity. However, no data on their long-term effects on weight loss and health is yet available.
5. *Potential development and worsening of eating disorders, and negative impact on their treatment.* GLP-1ARs, by increasing satiety, decreasing hunger, and in some people producing nausea, vomiting, and diarrhoea, can exacerbate extreme and rigid dietary restriction and the onset or worsening of eating disorder psychopathology [47]. Furthermore, the effects of GLP-1ARs on satiety/hunger could also negatively impact eating disorder treatments that require the intake of regular meals and snacks [47]. GLP-1ARs have not been approved for the treatment of any eating-disorder symptoms, and to date, information on misuse of these drugs has not yet been published. However, some authors have observed problematic use in their clinical practice [39], and warnings and calls to action regarding their potential misuse in adolescents with eating disorders have already been raised [47]. The current parenteral administration of the GLP-1RAs discourages their misuse, but when oral formulations become available, misuse will likely become a bigger issue [47].

The above data and considerations have led us to adopt a clinical stance on using GLP-1ARs in combination with CBT for patients with BED and clinical obesity. Specifically, we recommend that GLP-1ARs *not* be prescribed for the treatment of BED, or for reducing binge-eating episodes. Although some studies have reported a reduction in binge eating in patients with obesity without diabetes [28, 48], no data is available on the efficacy of GLP-1ARs in the treatment of BED, as the results of the only randomized control trial using liraglutide in this population were limited by the incorrect randomization of some participants [49]. Furthermore, it is suspected that their prescription in the initial phase of CBT for BED could exacerbate dysfunctional dieting and hinder the implementation of the regular eating procedure, a key and effective CBT strategy for addressing binge-eating episodes.

The exceptions to this general rule are patients with BED who are already taking these drugs for the management of type 2 diabetes or to control body weight, and need to continue their use. However, in such cases we stress that their use not be an obstacle to adopting the regular eating procedure or other procedures to address dysfunctional dieting.

In Step Two of the treatment, if the patient needs and wishes to lose a reasonable and healthy amount of weight but has difficulties in adhering to flexible and moderate dietary restriction, we weigh up with them the pros and cons of taking GLP-1ARs, as they are effective in the management of clinical obesity and its cardiometabolic complications. In these cases, we give detailed information to the patient on the downsides of GLP-1ARs, namely their side effects, cost, and the need for lifetime use. We emphasize the risk of adopting extreme dieting, which could promote the reactivation of binge-eating episodes and other features of eating-disorder psychopathology.

If a patient does elect to start medication, we ensure that they are periodically assessed by a physician who is an expert in managing clinical obesity, GLP-1AR drugs, and CBT principles for BED. We also advise associating these drugs with the healthy lifestyle modification described in this chapter. Indeed, healthy eating patterns and physical activity may offer additional benefits, enhancing the patient's health and well-being beyond weight loss alone [50].

References

1. Hagan KE, Forbush KT, Chen PY. Is dietary restraint a unitary or multi-faceted construct? Psychol Assess. 2017;29(10):1249–60. https://doi.org/10.1037/pas0000429.
2. Blomquist KK, Grilo CM. Predictive significance of changes in dietary restraint in obese patients with binge eating disorder during treatment. Int J Eat Disord. 2011;44(6):515–23. https://doi.org/10.1002/eat.20849.
3. Rueda-Clausen CF, Poddar M, Lear SA, Poirier P, Sharma AM. Canadian adult obesity clinical practice guidelines: assessment of people living with obesity. https://obesitycanada.ca/guidelines/assessment. (2020). Accessed.
4. Sharma AM. Does this person have obesity? EClinicalMedicine. 2023;58:101935. https://doi.org/10.1016/j.eclinm.2023.101935.
5. Estruch R, Ros E, Salas-Salvado J, Covas MI, Corella D, Aros F, et al. Primary prevention of cardiovascular disease with a mediterranean diet supplemented with extra-virgin olive oil or nut. N Engl J Med. 2018;378(25):e34. https://doi.org/10.1056/NEJMoa1800389.
6. Barry VW, Baruth M, Beets MW, Durstine JL, Liu J, Blair SN. Fitness vs. fatness on all-cause mortality: a meta-analysis. Prog Cardiovasc Dis. 2014;56(4):382–90. https://doi.org/10.1016/j.pcad.2013.09.002.
7. Barry VW, Caputo JL, Kang M. The joint association of fitness and fatness on cardiovascular disease mortality: a meta-analysis. Prog Cardiovasc Dis. 2018;61(2):136–41. https://doi.org/10.1016/j.pcad.2018.07.004.
8. Kroes M, Osei-Assibey G, Baker-Searle R, Huang J. Impact of weight change on quality of life in adults with overweight/obesity in the United States: a systematic review. Curr Med Res Opin. 2016;32(3):485–508. https://doi.org/10.1185/03007995.2015.1128403.
9. Jensen MD, Ryan DH, Apovian CM, Ard JD, Comuzzie AG, Donato KA, et al. AHA/ACC/TOS guideline for the management of overweight and obesity in adults: a report of the American College of Cardiology/American Heart Association task force on practice guidelines and the Obesity Society. J Am Coll Cardiol. 2014. 2013;63(25 Pt B):2985–3023. https://doi.org/10.1016/j.jacc.2013.11.004.
10. Knowler WC, Barrett-Connor E, Fowler SE, Hamman RF, Lachin JM, Walker EA, et al. Reduction in the incidence of type 2 diabetes with lifestyle intervention or metformin. N Engl J Med. 2002;346(6):393–403. https://doi.org/10.1056/NEJMoa012512.

11. Wing RR. Does lifestyle intervention improve health of adults with overweight/obesity and type 2 diabetes? Findings from the Look AHEAD randomized trial. Obesity. 2021;29(8):1246–58. https://doi.org/10.1002/oby.23158.
12. Tahrani AA, Morton J. Benefits of weight loss of 10% or more in patients with overweight or obesity: a review. Obesity. 2022;30(4):802–40. https://doi.org/10.1002/oby.23371.
13. Lean ME, Leslie WS, Barnes AC, Brosnahan N, Thom G, McCombie L, et al. Primary care-led weight management for remission of type 2 diabetes (DiRECT): an open-label, cluster-randomised trial. Lancet. 2018;391(10120):541–51. https://doi.org/10.1016/s0140-6736(17)33102-1.
14. Yurkow S, Ivezaj V, Grilo CM. Improvements in cardiovascular disease risk factors associated with modest weight loss following treatment in patients with binge-eating disorder and obesity. Int J Eat Disord. 2023;56(11):2074–83. https://doi.org/10.1002/eat.24035.
15. Dalle Grave R, Cuzzolaro M, Calugi S, Tomasi F, Temperilli F, Marchesini G. The effect of obesity management on body image in patients seeking treatment at medical centers. Obesity. 2007;15(9):2320–7.
16. Dalle Grave R, Calugi S, Gavasso I, El Ghoch M, Marchesini G. A randomized trial of energy-restricted high-protein versus high-carbohydrate, low-fat diet in morbid obesity. Obesity (Silver Spring). 2013;21(9):1774–81. https://doi.org/10.1002/oby.20320.
17. Horn DB, Almandoz JP, Look M. What is clinically relevant weight loss for your patients and how can it be achieved? A narrative review. Postgrad Med. 2022;134(4):359–75. https://doi.org/10.1080/00325481.2022.2051366.
18. Schwarzfuchs D, Golan R, Shai I. Four-year follow-up after two-year dietary interventions. N Engl J Med. 2012;367(14):1373–4. https://doi.org/10.1056/NEJMc1204792.
19. Gotsis E, Anagnostis P, Mariolis A, Vlachou A, Katsiki N, Karagiannis A. Health benefits of the Mediterranean diet: an update of research over the last 5 years. Angiology. 2015;66(4):304–18. https://doi.org/10.1177/0003319714532169.
20. Dalle Grave R, Sartirana M, El Ghoch M, Calugi S. Treating obesity with personalized cognitive behavioral therapy. Cham: Springer; 2018.
21. Wheeler ML, Franz M, Barrier P, Holler H, Cronmiller N, Delahanty LM. Macronutrient and energy database for the 1995 exchange lists for meal planning: a rationale for clinical practice decisions. J Am Diet Assoc. 1996;96(11):1167–71. https://doi.org/10.1016/s0002-8223(96)00299-4.
22. FAO/WHO/UNU. Human energy requirements. Report of a joint FAO/WHO/UNU expert consultation. Rome: FAO: food and nutrition technical report series 1; 2004.
23. Hollands GJ, Shemilt I, Marteau TM, Jebb SA, Lewis HB, Wei Y, et al. Portion, package or tableware size for changing selection and consumption of food, alcohol and tobacco. Cochrane Database Syst Rev. 2015;2015(9):Cd011045. https://doi.org/10.1002/14651858.CD011045.pub2.
24. Sacks FM, Bray GA, Carey VJ, Smith SR, Ryan DH, Anton SD, et al. Comparison of weight-loss diets with different compositions of fat, protein, and carbohydrates. N Engl J Med. 2009;360(9):859–73. https://doi.org/10.1056/NEJMoa0804748.
25. Widmer RJ, Flammer AJ, Lerman LO, Lerman A. The Mediterranean diet, its components, and cardiovascular disease. Am J Med. 2015;128(3):229–38. https://doi.org/10.1016/j.amjmed.2014.10.014.
26. Burke LE, Wang J, Sevick MA. Self-monitoring in weight loss: a systematic review of the literature. J Am Diet Assoc. 2011;111(1):92–102. https://doi.org/10.1016/j.jada.2010.10.008.
27. Gamble JM, Clarke A, Myers KJ, Agnew MD, Hatch K, Snow MM, et al. Incretin-based medications for type 2 diabetes: an overview of reviews. Diabetes Obes Metab. 2015;17(7):649–58. https://doi.org/10.1111/dom.12465.
28. Chao AM, Tronieri JS, Amaro A, Wadden TA. Semaglutide for the treatment of obesity. Trends Cardiovasc Med. 2023;33(3):159–66. https://doi.org/10.1016/j.tcm.2021.12.008.
29. Pi-Sunyer X, Astrup A, Fujioka K, Greenway F, Halpern A, Krempf M, et al. A randomized, controlled trial of 3.0 mg of Liraglutide in weight management. N Engl J Med. 2015;373(1):11–22. https://doi.org/10.1056/NEJMoa1411892.

30. Wharton S, Batterham RL, Bhatta M, Buscemi S, Christensen LN, Frias JP, et al. Two-year effect of semaglutide 2.4 mg on control of eating in adults with overweight/obesity: STEP 5. Obesity. 2023;31(3):703–15. https://doi.org/10.1002/oby.23673.
31. Friedrichsen M, Breitschaft A, Tadayon S, Wizert A, Skovgaard D. The effect of semaglutide 2.4 mg once weekly on energy intake, appetite, control of eating, and gastric emptying in adults with obesity. Diabetes Obes Metab. 2021;23(3):754–62. https://doi.org/10.1111/dom.14280.
32. Heise T, DeVries JH, Urva S, Li J, Pratt EJ, Thomas MK, et al. Tirzepatide reduces appetite, energy intake, and fat mass in people with type 2 diabetes. Diabetes Care. 2023;46(5):998–1004. https://doi.org/10.2337/dc22-1710.
33. Jastreboff AM, Aronne LJ, Ahmad NN, Wharton S, Connery L, Alves B, et al. Tirzepatide once weekly for the treatment of obesity. N Engl J Med. 2022. https://doi.org/10.1056/NEJMoa2206038.
34. Lincoff AM, Brown-Frandsen K, Colhoun HM, Deanfield J, Emerson SS, Esbjerg S, et al. Semaglutide and cardiovascular outcomes in obesity without diabetes. N Engl J Med. 2023;389(24):2221–32. https://doi.org/10.1056/NEJMoa2307563.
35. Butler J, Abildstrøm SZ, Borlaug BA, Davies MJ, Kitzman DW, Petrie MC, et al. Semaglutide in patients with obesity and heart failure across mildly reduced or preserved ejection fraction. J Am Coll Cardiol. 2023;82(22):2087–96. https://doi.org/10.1016/j.jacc.2023.09.811.
36. Malhotra A, Grunstein RR, Fietze I, Weaver TE, Redline S, Azarbarzin A, et al. Tirzepatide for the treatment of obstructive sleep Apnea and obesity. N Engl J Med. 2024. https://doi.org/10.1056/NEJMoa2404881.
37. Food and Drug Administration (FDA): Wegovy (semaglutide) injection prescribing information. https://www.accessdata.fda.gov/drugsatfda_docs/label/2023/215256s007lbl.pdf (2023). Accessed.
38. Sodhi M, Rezaeianzadeh R, Kezouh A, Etminan M. Risk of gastrointestinal adverse events associated with glucagon-like Peptide-1 receptor agonists for weight loss. JAMA. 2023; https://doi.org/10.1001/jama.2023.19574.
39. Bartel S, McElroy SL, Levangie D, Keshen A. Use of glucagon-like peptide-1 receptor agonists in eating disorder populations. Int J Eat Disord. 2023; https://doi.org/10.1002/eat.24109.
40. Wadden TA, Chao AM, Moore M, Tronieri JS, Gilden A, Amaro A, et al. The role of lifestyle modification with second-generation anti-obesity medications: comparisons, questions, and clinical opportunities. Curr Obes Rep. 2023;12(4):453–73. https://doi.org/10.1007/s13679-023-00534-z.
41. Zamboni M, Rubele S, Rossi AP. Sarcopenia and obesity. Curr Opin Clin Nutr Metab Care. 2019;22(1):13–9. https://doi.org/10.1097/mco.0000000000000519.
42. Chaston TB, Dixon JB, O'Brien PE. Changes in fat-free mass during significant weight loss: a systematic review. Int J Obes. 2007;31(5):743–50. https://doi.org/10.1038/sj.ijo.0803483.
43. Wilding JPH, Batterham RL, Calanna S, Davies M, Van Gaal LF, Lingvay I, et al. Once-weekly semaglutide in adults with overweight or obesity. N Engl J Med. 2021;384(11):989. https://doi.org/10.1056/NEJMoa2032183.
44. Do D, Lee T, Peasah SK, Good CB, Inneh A, Patel U. GLP-1 receptor agonist discontinuation among patients with obesity and/or type 2 diabetes. JAMA Netw Open. 2024;7(5). https://doi.org/10.1001/jamanetworkopen.2024.13172.
45. Wilding JPH, Batterham RL, Davies M, Van Gaal LF, Kandler K, Konakli K, et al. Weight regain and cardiometabolic effects after withdrawal of semaglutide: the STEP 1 trial extension. Diabetes Obes Metab. 2022;24(8):1553–64. https://doi.org/10.1111/dom.14725.
46. Aronne LJ, Sattar N, Horn DB, Bays HE, Wharton S, Lin WY, et al. Continued treatment with Tirzepatide for maintenance of weight reduction in adults with obesity: the SURMOUNT-4 randomized clinical trial. JAMA. 2023. https://doi.org/10.1001/jama.2023.24945.
47. Cooper DM, Rothstein MA, Amin A, Hirsch JD, Cooper E. Unintended consequences of glucagon-like peptide-1 receptor agonists medications in children and adolescents: a call to action. J Clin Transl Sci. 2023;7(1):e184. https://doi.org/10.1017/cts.2023.612.

48. Robert SA, Rohana AG, Shah SA, Chinna K, Wan Mohamud WN, Kamaruddin NA. Improvement in binge eating in non-diabetic obese individuals after 3 months of treatment with liraglutide—a pilot study. Obes Res Clin Pract. 2015;9(3):301–4. https://doi.org/10.1016/j.orcp.2015.03.005.
49. Allison KC, Chao AM, Bruzas MB, McCuen-Wurst C, Jones E, McAllister C, et al. A pilot randomized controlled trial of liraglutide 3.0 mg for binge eating disorder. Obes Sci Pract. 2023;9(2):127–36. https://doi.org/10.1002/osp4.619.
50. Dalle GR. The benefit of healthy lifestyle in the era of new medications to treat obesity. Diabetes Metab Syndr Obes. 2024;17:227–30. https://doi.org/10.2147/dmso.S447582.

Events, Moods, and Eating Module 13

Abstract

This module is indicated for patients in whom events and associated moods contribute to the maintenance of binge-eating episodes and other types of dysfunctional eating. This mechanism is recognizable because it leads to repeated deviations from regular eating associated with events or changes in mood. Predictable events influencing eating are addressed via the proactive problem-solving procedure, and unpredictable events via the procedure of things to say (also known as urge surfing) and do (also known as alternative activities). In the subgroup of patients who are highly sensitive to any intense mood state and manage emotional changes through dysfunctional mood-modulation behaviours (e.g., alcohol or substance misuse, self-harm, binge eating), the module introduces specific strategies and procedures to intervene in the sequence of events leading to mood intolerance and deploy functional mood-modulation behaviours. The module is also indicated for patients with binge-eating disorder (BED) using binge eating as their primary source of reward in life. In such cases, patients are helped to identify rewarding activities and their consequences, and to increase the importance of other rewarding activities. Finally, the module also includes the procedure of binge-eating analysis to help the patient address residual binge-eating episodes.

Events and associated changes in mood often influence the eating behaviour of individuals with BED. This association becomes more apparent as treatment progresses, especially as major mechanisms maintaining binge-eating episodes (e.g., dysregulated eating and dysfunctional dieting) are eliminated. Typical mood-related changes in eating include dysregulated eating, overeating, and binge eating. The main mechanisms responsible for this association are as follows [1]:

- Eating is used to distract from adverse events and from problems that cause concerns

R. Dalle Grave et al., *Cognitive Behavior Therapy for Binge Eating Disorder*,
https://doi.org/10.1007/978-3-031-71456-6_13

- Eating is used to mitigate intense and intolerable emotional states
- Eating is used as a source of reward

13.1 Assessing Whether Events and Moods Warrant Addressing

In Step Two, it is important to determine whether events and moods are contributing to maintaining binge-eating episodes and other types of dysfunctional eating. If so, the patient should be assisted in addressing them directly and effectively. This mechanism is recognizable because it leads to repeated deviations from regular eating associated with events or changes in mood, as evidenced by the patient's monitoring records. Deviations may manifest as recurrent binge-eating episodes, dysregulated eating, or overeating.

13.2 Addressing Predictable Events Influencing Eating

First, CBT for BED addresses predictable events influencing eating via the proactive problem-solving procedure. A predictable event is a situation that is expected to increase the risk of deviating from the food plan (e.g., being invited to a dinner with friends or attending a wedding lunch), or one that is repeatedly associated with binge-eating episodes, dysregulated eating, and/or overeating (e.g., eating while cooking, binge eating at a particular hour of the day).

To train the patient to use proactive problem-solving, the therapist should first identify a recent episode of a deviation from planned eating related to an event. Possible triggers for "emotional eating" include boredom, interpersonal difficulties and work pressure, as well as adverse emotional states. Once identified, the therapist and the patient should seek to reconstruct the sequence of the triggering event and subsequent thoughts, feelings and behaviours. Then, the therapist should help the patient see that this sequence could have been interrupted, and help them understand where. The goal is to introduce the concept that such changes in eating are not inevitable. For example, the sequence of events could have been interrupted by a friend's phone call inviting the patient to go out. Using this example, we teach the patient how to use the proactive problem-solving procedure to address similar events that trigger changes in eating. The procedure we use involves seven steps:

Step One: Identifying the problem as early on as possible. Every time an adverse event could lead to a change in eating, patients should try to identify the underlying problem.

Step Two: Accurately specifying the problem. It is often not easy to understand the true nature of the problem: many people initially say that they simply feel an automatic urge to binge, more powerful than their ability to resist. In reality, careful analysis often reveals that the real issue is not bingeing but an inability to handle boredom, loneliness, or interpersonal conflicts, for example.

Step Three: Considering a range of possible solutions. The third step is to think of as many potential solutions to the problem as possible (brainstorming), no matter how nonsensical or impractical they seem. Even implausible solutions should be included on the list, as this may lead to a solution or suggestion that would otherwise not be thought of.

Step Four: Thinking through the implications of each solution. This is a critical step in which the patient is asked to weigh the pros and cons of each potential solution.

Step Five: Choosing the best solution(s). This should be easy if the previous step has been completed carefully.

Step Six: Putting the best solution(s) into practice. The crucial point of the problem-solving process is to *act* and apply the chosen solution(s). Patients should be instructed not to be too inflexible in adhering to what they have planned: if they notice that the selected solution is not sufficiently effective, they should try another of the potential solutions identified in Steps Three and Four of the process.

Step Seven: Assessing the process of problem-solving. The last step is to review the entire process afterward, perhaps the next day, to understand if it could have been done better. The most important thing is not to evaluate whether the problem has been solved, even though this is relevant, but whether the problem-solving could have been done better. In the next session, the patient and therapist should discuss the entire process together, and if necessary, work together on finding ways to improve the procedure.

Once the proactive problem-solving procedure has been practiced in-session, the patient is asked to identify and address problems proactively, i.e., before they happen, as homework. To do this, the patient is encouraged to reflect on what events could trigger changes in their eating, and think about how to address them using the proactive problem-solving procedure. Specifically, once the patient identifies a potentially risky event, they should write "PROBLEM" in the Comments column of their monitoring record and, on its back, draft the first six steps of the procedure. The therapist should encourage using this tool whenever necessary, and advise the patient to write down the procedure rather than do it mentally to make it more effective. Figure 13.1 shows an example of the proactive problem-solving procedure performed by a patient.

When asked if they have identified any problems to solve, some patients say that they have no problems to solve. In such cases, we emphasize that everyone faces problems more or less every day. Examples can be identified by examining their monitoring records for the preceding week. We encourage patients to practice the proactive problem-solving procedure, even for more minor difficulties, so that they can handle more significant ones when they arise.

Step 1: When I'm home alone in the afternoon, I binge eat.

Step 2: I tend to binge in the afternoon around 6 when I'm alone doing homework and feeling bored.

Step 3: Solutions	*Step 4: Pros (+) and Cons (-)*
	+ It keeps me away from food, relaxes me *- It's raining*
Chat with friends	*+ Can help me relax, and I don't feel lonely* *- Not always possible*
Urge surf the impulse to binge	*+ It's about time I handle the impulse without binging* *- I am afraid of succumbing as usual to the impulse to binge*
Do my nails	*+ It's something I enjoy* *- I can only do it occasionally*
Have a snack a bit later	*+ It's a good idea,so I don't come home hungry* *- None*

Step 5: What are the solutions that can be helpful?
Doing my nails, and having a snack later.

Step 6: On Thursday, I had a snack around 5:30, then took half an hour to do my nails. I managed not to binge."

Step 7: Next time, in addition to having a snack later, I could spend some time chatting with my friend and practicing urge surfing the impulse to binge. Anyway, it went well.

Fig. 13.1 Example of a proactive problem-solving by a patient with BED

13.3 Addressing Sudden Events Influencing Eating

If applied proactively, the problem-solving procedure helps prevent mood changes due to predictable events. However, adverse emotional states can also be triggered by unpredictable events or circumstances. For this reason, it is necessary for the patient to be forearmed with strategies for changing mood without changing eating behaviour. We suggest, in addition to real-time monitoring, encouraging the patient to practice applying the "things to say and do" strategy (see Sect. 8.3.5 and the example in Table 8.2), which was introduced in Step One of the treatment to improve their adherence to the regular eating procedure. In this case too, the patient should preventatively fill in and keep to hand a "coping card" that they can consult when they start to feel overwhelmed.

13.4 Addressing Mood Intolerance

Some individuals with BED are susceptible to any intense mood state, and manage emotional changes through dysfunctional mood-modulation behaviours (e.g., alcohol or substance misuse, self-harm, binge-eating episodes) that help neutralize or reduce awareness of emotions. However, such behaviours are harmful and, more importantly, do not help in a patient to learn healthy ways to manage mood states. The presence of mood intolerance should be suspected if the patient reports a recurring association between mood changes and certain behavioural expressions of eating disorders, and if proactive problem-solving and things to say and do have not been sufficient to manage the problem. If this is the case, the procedures described in the following paragraphs may be helpful.

13.4.1 Providing Personalized Education Mood Intolerance

If the therapist suspects the presence of mood intolerance, they should discuss with the patient its role in maintaining binge-eating episodes, adding it to the personal formulation and assessing the need to address it. It should be explained to the patient that some mood-modulation behaviours, including binge-eating episodes, are dysfunctional because, while helping them to cope with mood changes in the short-term, they are a harmful substitute for the acquisition of the skills needed to manage mood changes effectively. The therapist should warn the patient that learning to tolerate emotions more functionally will be challenging but worthwhile.

13.4.2 Analyzing a Recent Example of Mood Intolerance

The therapist should analyze with the patient a recent example of mood intolerance to recreate the sequence of seven events [2]:

1. Triggering event (e.g., an argument with their partner)
2. Cognitive appraisal of the event (e.g., "*He doesn't understand me, he always blames me.*")
3. Secondary mood change (e.g., anger)
4. Cognitive evaluation of mood change, with rapid amplification of emotion intensity (e.g., "*I can't stand this anger, I feel terrible; I CAN'T STAND THIS ANGER, I FEEL TERRIBLE;* ***I CAN'T STAND THIS ANGER, I FEEL TERRIBLE!***")
5. Dysfunctional mood modulation behaviour (e.g., alcohol intake and binge eating)
6. Short-term improvement in mood state
7. Later cognitive appraisal (e.g., "*I have no self-control/I'm a failure/I disgust myself/I'll never recover from my eating problem/I'm addicted to food.*")

13.4.3 Understanding the Mechanisms Involved in Mood Intolerance

Next, the therapist should educate the patient about the processes involved in mood intolerance, emphasizing two points:

1. Each episode consists of a rapid sequence of thoughts and emotions that prompt the dysfunctional mood-modulation behaviour.
2. New areas of intervention emerge if the chain of events can be slowed down and analyzed.

13.4.4 Slowing Down and Analyzing the Sequence of Thoughts and Emotions

The patient should be encouraged to capture the sequence of thoughts and emotions the next time they experience an impulse to adopt dysfunctional emotion-modulation behaviour, or immediately afterward, writing it down as soon as possible on the back of their monitoring record. The patient should be forewarned that the procedure may be frustrating because it prevents them "escaping" from the adverse mood state, but if continued, will increase awareness of the sequence of events and, by slowing it down, help prevent cognitive amplification and present ideas of where to intervene and "stop the train in its tracks".

13.4.5 Intervening in the Sequence of Events

The next step is to suggest procedures for the patient to apply at various points in the sequence of events.

Preventing the triggering event. If the event is predictable, the patient is advised to use the proactive problem-solving procedure, which can help thwart most mood-intolerance episodes.

Cognitive appraisal of events. The use of cognitive restructuring can help the patient interpret events more functionally. In particular, the patient should be helped to restructure "all-or-nothing" thoughts and negative global assessments of the event, and come to a less extreme and negative conclusion. Additionally, the patient should conduct behavioural experiments to test their new interpretation of events.

Accepting emotions. The patient should be educated about emotions in general, and the following concepts in particular: (i) emotions are part of normal human experience, and there is nothing wrong with feeling sad or anxious at times; (ii) emotions rarely persist for a long time unless a person has depression or an anxiety disorder; and (iii) it is useful to understand the emotional state and label it (e.g., anger, anxiety, sadness). Awareness of the physical experiences associated with emotions can help understand the emotion experienced (e.g., muscle tension = anxiety; boiling blood sensation = anger; weariness = sadness). It is also important not to confuse thoughts (e.g., I feel like a failure) with emotions (e.g., sadness), and to discern the associated mood state. The next step is to encourage the patient to accept the emotion without reacting; emphasize that with this procedure they will observe the emotion wax, wane, and then fade away (the "emotion wave" concept). This is a good way of debunking the belief that negative emotions will continue to worsen until a dysfunctional behaviour is adopted to modulate them. The patient is also encouraged to pay attention to thoughts that amplify the emotion (e.g., "*I can't bear being in this state*", "*It's terrible to feel this emotion*", "*If I don't do something, it'll keep getting worse*", "*I absolutely must do something calm this mood*".). A strategy to curb cognitive amplification of emotions is to write them down on the monitoring record as they occur.

13.4.6 Using Functional Mood-Modulation Behaviours

When the patient experiences a mood change, they should adopt functional mood-modulation behaviours such as listening to happy music if they are sad or relaxing music if they are angry or stressed, communicating with others, or taking a brisk walk, a relaxing bath, or a cold shower. Initially, these behaviours are less effective in changing the mood state than dysfunctional ones. However, their effectiveness increases over time, and they have the advantage of not producing negative consequences.

Success in using functional emotion-modulation behaviours helps to change a patient's beliefs that their mood state is out of control and can only be managed by dysfunctional behaviours (e.g., "*Only food can help me reduce my anxiety.*"). It is also crucial for the patient to try to lessen the chances of dysfunctional mood-modulation behaviours by eliminating any psychoactive substances or tools (e.g., alcohol, drugs, razors or other utensils) usually used for dysfunctional coping strategies.

Vignette

The patient, a 25-year-old woman, has daily binge-eating episodes not followed by compensatory behaviours and occasional episodes of excessive alcohol intake. These behaviours, which started at the age of 17, one month after an episode of sexual assault by a peer, led to a weight gain of about 30 kg in a year (from 54 to 84 kg). In the following years, to try to lose the weight she had gained, she intermittently adopted extreme and rigid dietary rules (skipping meals and eliminating many foods), which were interrupted by binge-eating episodes. These behaviours were associated with a progressive weight gain up to a maximum weight of 98 kg at the time of the first assessment at our centre.

The patient appreciated CBT for BED immediately, mainly its focus on addressing binge eating first, and got actively engaged in treatment. In Step One, she succeeded in regulating her eating after a couple of weeks, having three meals plus two snacks a day, and significantly reduced the frequency of binge-eating episodes, from several times a day to one or two times a week, with no episodes of alcohol intake. She also increased her number of daily steps.

In Step Two, she decided to focus only on the eating disorder, not her weight, and an analysis of residual binge-eating episodes highlighted that these were often triggered by rapid mood changes. For this reason, it was decided, in agreement with the patient, to address mood intolerance because the proactive problem-solving procedure had proven insufficient to manage them. The procedures allowed the patient to interrupt binge-eating episodes in a few weeks and understand that she could tolerate mood changes by accepting and managing them more functionally (e.g., by listening to a podcast and taking a walk).

13.5 Addressing the Use of Binge Eating as a Reward

Some patients with BED use binge eating as their primary source of reward in life. Perceiving the positive aspects of binge-eating episodes, they are reluctant to stop them completely. In such cases, first and foremost, we explore with the patient the advantages they perceive from binge eating (e.g., immediate enjoyment of eating, and a sense of well-being). Subsequently, we analyze the disadvantages (e.g., potential weight gain, money spent, secrecy and deception, subsequent self-criticism, and eating disorder maintenance). A detailed analysis of the pros and cons can help the patient fully realize the short-term and long-term costs of binge eating, making them more open to using the strategies described below, which are designed to help interrupt such episodes.

13.5.1 Identify Rewarding Activities and Their Consequences

This topic should be introduced by discussing with the patient that the need for reward is a fundamental element in anyone's life. The patient should then be assisted in identifying their specific "rewarding activities", and drawing them on a pie chart, where the size of each slice represents the degree of gratification obtained from each rewarding activity (the larger the slice, the more gratifying the activity). The implications of their pie chart should be discussed, and a plan should be devised to address any problems associated with using food as the primary form of reward. The following is an example of dialogue between a therapist and a patient addressing the use of binge eating as a reward:

Therapist: So, looking at the course of your treatment, it seems increasingly clear that we have identified an important mechanism maintaining your binge-eating episodes.

Patient: Yes, I realize that food is an important part of my life.

Therapist: I agree. Food seems to be a significant source of gratification in your life.

Patient: Exactly: if I think I can't eat what I like, or enjoy new and special foods, my day is ruined. After all, food is the spice of life!

Therapist: Certainly! Food is one of life's great pleasures. However, I would like to discuss whether other things make you happy. Everyone is seeking gratification. It drives us forward, even if the day has been rather dull or stressful. For example, some people find satisfaction in pursuing a hobby, like photography; others are gratified by their work, and some get their sense of reward from engaging in a sport, buying new clothes or gifts, or simply chatting with friends. Of course, as we said, food is very gratifying, but many people engage in various rewarding activities, not just eating, allowing them to derive more pleasure from life. Don't you agree?

Patient: Yes, I do.

Therapist: So, I think we should explore what other options you have. We need to consider three parameters to understand whether an activity is rewarding. The first is your desire to do it, the second is the pleasure you experience while doing it, and the third is the frustration you feel if you can't do it. Clear?

Patient: Yes, I think so. For example, a colleague of mine can't wait to get home to build his model aeroplanes: it's his passion.

Therapist: Exactly! I'm sure building model aeroplanes is a rewarding activity for him. Now let's figure out what your rewarding activities are at this stage of your life. A good way to represent them is to draw a pie chart, in which each slice represents activities you perceive as rewarding, and the size of each slice reflects how gratifying you find them. Before we start, however, I suggest you list of all the activities you find rewarding.

The therapist helps the patient generate a list of rewarding activities. If the patient has difficulty identifying rewards other than food, the therapist should explain that rewarding activities may have become part of their life without them being consciously aware of them. To clarify what these activities are, the therapist should ask the patient to focus on their typical days to determine if interrupting certain routine activities—such as taking a coffee break with colleagues, taking a child to school, or listening to music in the car—would cause frustration and a general reduction in daily satisfaction. The more examples the therapist provides, the easier it will be for the patient to recognize some of their rewarding activities.

Once the list of rewarding activities has been created, the therapist should draw the pie chart under the patient's direction: the more rewarding an activity, the larger the corresponding slice. The patient should be told that the best way to understand the size of the slice representing the rewarding activity is to think about the intensity and duration of frustration when they cannot engage in it—the more frustrating its absence, the larger the slice should be. The therapist should then ask the patient for their opinion on the pie chart.

Figure 13.2 shows an example of a dysfunctional pie chart dominated by a large slice representing reward obtained from food, accompanied by a few other, less rewarding activities, and a functional pie chart with a greater number of rewarding

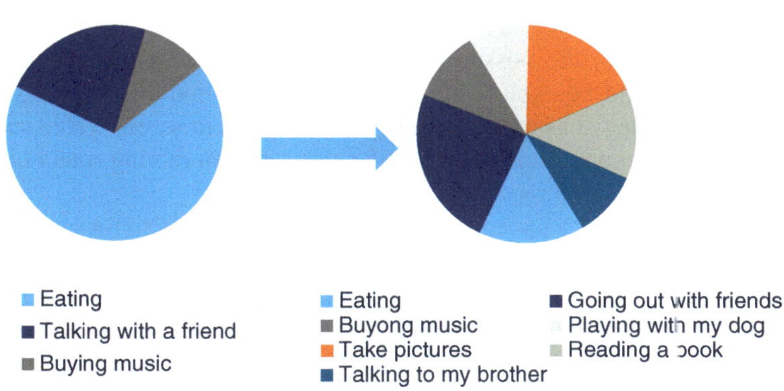

Fig. 13.2 A dysfunctional pie chart (left) and a functional pie chart (right) of rewarding activities

activities and no predominant one. Many patients whose pie chart is like the former are embarrassed and ashamed of the importance they attribute to food. They should, however, be reassured that this is common to many people and is something they can change.

As a homework assignment, the patient should be encouraged to review their pie chart daily, and consider whether it accurately represents the true state of their rewarding activities based on that day's attitudes and behaviours. It might be helpful for the patient to redraw the pie chart at the end of each day (on the back of the monitoring record). In the next session, these should be further discussed and redrawn, with the size of the slices being adjusted as needed.

Once the pie chart has been created, the therapist should discuss with the patient the implications of their rewarding activities and encourage them to think if they may pose a problem. This discussion should identify the main negative consequences of using food as the primary form of gratification. At this stage, the therapist should explain to the patient that having a pie chart with a dominant slice can be risky. This is because gratification rests predominantly on a single activity, everything may seem fine as long as that activity can be practiced. However, when, for some reason, it cannot, life seems less meaningful and satisfying. Another problem with having a pie chart dominated by a single slice is that this narrow interest is self-perpetuating and marginalizes other activities. As a result, interests, attitudes and relationships can be reduced to situations in which food must be present. Finally, if the predominant rewarding activity, such as binge eating, is practiced excessively, it can have negative health consequences and serve as a factor promoting the onset and maintenance of eating disorder and clinical obesity (see Sect. 4.3.1 and Table 4.4 for the definition).

13.5.2 Increasing the Importance of Other Rewarding Activities

Once the patient becomes aware of the importance of addressing binge eating as the primary form of reward, two strategies can be adopted. First, the patient should be encouraged to break the link between seeking pleasure and binge eating by using the procedures previously described for managing predictable events (proactive problem-solving). Next, the possibility of obtaining gratification from activities other than food should be explored and encouraged. It should be emphasized to patients that this strategy has the advantage of making life more enjoyable, creating and maintaining new opportunities for gratification, and not relying solely on binging as the primary source of reward.

The first step in helping a patient engage in other rewarding activities is to explain the rationale behind it. For example, the therapist might say, "*We know that effectively managing your eating and weight is an important goal in your life. However, together we have noticed that you often seek gratification through food, which is a significant obstacle to managing your weight. One way to address this obstacle is to engage in other rewarding activities. Investing time in other activities will allow you to discover that food is just one of many rewarding activities and may be the least helpful for you.*"

The second step should be to identify new pleasurable activities that the patient might be interested in. Clues to these activities may come from past hobbies or interests that the patient used to pursue but has abandoned, and/or considering what their friends or colleagues do in their free time. At this stage, a "brainstorming" approach is best, creating a list of all possibilities, even if they seem (to the patient) silly or intimidating. If a patient reports not having time for other activities because they are too busy with family and work, etc., the therapist should remind them that to achieve success in effectively managing their eating and weight, it is essential for them to consider treatment a priority, and finding new sources of reward could be a crucial step in this process.

The third step involves agreeing on one or two pleasurable activities that the patient will try to include in their life. These can be anything as long as they are feasible and habitual. The patient should involve other people (especially significant others) in these activities, and it should be a decision in which they feel engaged, making it more likely that they stick with it over time.

Once the patient has agreed to engage in a new pleasurable activity, the fourth step is to ensure that they start doing it. The therapist should ask the patient to use the last column of their monitoring record to document this activity, and any obstacles they encounter while doing it. These should be reviewed later, and appropriate solutions sought. The therapist should not be shy about actively encouraging the hesitant patient to start. For example, if the patient is considering enrolling in a photography course, it would be appropriate for the therapist to help them find suitable courses and discuss enrolment procedures. Getting the patient started should be the main priority at this stage. The patient's progress should be reviewed weekly (as a fixed item on the session agenda), and the therapist should encourage and facilitate adherence. The patient should be helped to use the proactive problem-solving procedure to overcome any difficulties. It is important to note that rewarding activities can change during treatment, as unsuitable ones may be eliminated, and additional activities may be identified and adopted.

Vignette

A 35-year-old single patient reported finding eating extremely rewarding, and that when binge-eating, she experienced intense pleasure. She also mentioned that after a long day at work, she usually found herself thinking: "*What's better than eating? Just the thought makes me feel good!*". Understandably, the patient had difficulty giving up this habit because, even though she recognized it as an obstacle to resolving her eating problem, she thought she would feel deprived without this source of reward. However, with the therapist's help, the patient identified two alternative evening activities that did not involve eating that could be rewarding: reading her favourite books and attending a film club.

Although not without some initial difficulties, the patient learned to see the benefit of her new "hobbies", which she enjoyed and allowed her to make new friends.

13.6 Addressing Residual Binge Episodes

The regular eating procedure introduced in Step One is an effective intervention for addressing binge-eating episodes, and is sufficient to interrupt them in some patients. However, with other patients, binge-eating episodes persist even during Step Two, albeit with reduced frequency. In such cases, they are called "residual binge-eating episodes". Analyzing these episodes can help shed light on the processes that contribute to them and allow them to be addressed through specific procedures.

13.6.1 Binge Analysis

Binge-eating analysis is a strategy for helping the patient address residual binge-eating episodes. The first step is to explain to the patient that episodes are not sudden and inexplicable, but rather the product of one or more of five well-defined processes [2]:

1. Breaking a dietary rule and then reacting by temporarily abandoning control over eating.
2. Dysfunctional undereating. Some patients persistently or intermittently maintain a highly calorie-restricted diet and tend to delay eating during the day, thus being under intense biological pressure to eat later on.
3. Using food as a reward.
4. Adverse events and associated mood changes that trigger overeating.
5. Consumption of alcohol or other psychoactive substances that cause disinhibition and make it harder to maintain control over eating.

After the therapist has explained these five processes to the patient, they should encourage the patient to see each subsequent binge-eating episode as an "interesting phenomenon" that can be studied to learn which of the five processes was behind it (there may be more than one) and what they can take from this to prevent future occurrences. [2]. Analyzing each binge-eating episode has two important effects:

1. It counters the patient's tendency to feel overwhelmed and demoralized after a binge, and their attribution of their loss of control to a lack of self-control: a reaction that risks triggering a subsequent episode.
2. It enables the selection and deployment of specific procedures that can increase the likelihood of eliminating residual binge episodes.

   Specific procedures for addressing the five main processes maintaining binge-eating episodes are as follows:

- Breaking a dietary rule: continue addressing cognitive dietary restraint (see Chap. 14).

- Dysfunctional undereating: continue addressing extreme and rigid dietary restriction (see Chap. 14).
- Adverse events and associated mood changes: use the proactive problem-solving procedure and reconsider incorporating procedures to address mood intolerance.
- Using food as a reward: use the procedures described in Sect. 13.4.
- Consumption of alcohol or other psychoactive substances: psychoeducation and support intervention.

References

1. Dalle Grave R, Calugi S. Cognitive behavior therapy for adolescents with eating disorders. New York: Guilford Press; 2020.
2. Fairburn CG. Cognitive behavior therapy and eating disorders. New York: Guilford Press; 2008.

Dysfunctional Dieting Module 14

Abstract

The module is indicated for patients with a persistent dysfunctional diet characterized by extreme and rigid dietary rules. This eating pattern causes profound harm and is one of the main mechanisms maintaining binge-eating episodes. To help them overcome dysfunctional dieting, patients are first helped to see it as a problem, then to identify and address their dietary rules (e.g., food avoidance, how much to eat, not eating in front of others, eating less than others present, not eating unless hungry, not eating unless earned, avoiding eating at restaurants, pizzerias, fast food joints, and buffets), and dysfunctional reactions to dietary rule violations, using specific cognitive behavior (CBT) strategies and procedures.

It is not uncommon for some individuals with BED and clincal obesity (see Sect. 4.3.1 and Table 4.4 for the definition), especially those who have overvaluation of shape and weight and/or unrealistic weight goals, to adopt a persistent and highly distinctive and dysfunctional form of dieting when they try to lose weight. Instead of following flexible general guidelines on when, how much, and what to eat, they adhere to specific dietary rules to restrict their food intake [1]. This module targets such dysfunctional dieting, which has three main characteristics [2]: (i) it is persistent; (ii) it has extreme goals (i.e., characterized by many dietary rules requiring continuous monitoring and constant commitment), and (iii) it has rigid dietary rules (i.e., the dietary rules must be followed perfectly to maintain a feeling of being in control). This type of diet is primarily motivated by the desire to rapidly lose a significant amount of weight and/or to modify body shape and/or to maintain strict control over food intake.

Dietary rules may vary from person to person, but generally involve when to eat (e.g., never having breakfast and snacks), how much to eat (e.g., fewer than

R. Dalle Grave et al., *Cognitive Behavior Therapy for Binge Eating Disorder*, https://doi.org/10.1007/978-3-031-71456-6_14

1,000 kcal per day), and what to eat (e.g., "food avoidance": avoiding a large number of foods, especially carbohydrates). The consequence is that eating becomes stereotyped and inflexible. It is important to distinguish between two aspects of dysfunctional dieting:

1. Extreme and rigid dietary restraint: an attempt to limit food intake by adopting rigid and extreme dietary rules.
2. Severe calorie restriction: an extreme reduction in daily calorie intake (e.g., below 1,200 kcal per day).

Dysfunctional dieting causes profound harm to those who attempt to adhere to either extreme and rigid dietary restraint or severe calorie restriction, to the point where everyday eating becomes an extremely anxiety-inducing experience marked by deep feelings of guilt. Consequently, social eating is heavily impacted, with individuals avoiding situations where food is involved.

To address dysfunctional dieting, we adopt a dual strategy. The first involves focusing on the motivations that drive its implementation, particularly concerns about weight and body shape, and working towards seeing them as problematic. The second entails changing eating behaviours.

14.1 Helping the Patient See Dysfunctional Dieting as a Problem

One of the main obstacles in addressing the dysfunctional diet is that the patient often does not perceive it as a problem for several reasons [3]:

- It creates a strong sense of control.
- It is a way to manage weight and body shape.
- It is socially reinforced.
- Some individuals perceive themselves as skilled in following it, viewing it as a measure of their willpower: if they fail to adhere, they feel guilty or weak.
- The diet is a primary means of compensation for individuala with binge-eating episodes.
- People with clinical obesity often perceive it as a necessary means of managing their higher weight.

Therefore, the first step in addressing dysfunctional dieting is helping the patient to recognize it as a problem. To do this, the therapist should discuss with them the two following points:

1. The diet is a problem if it is "rigid," i.e., characterized by specific dietary rules that must be followed perfectly to feel in control. This type of diet promotes binge-eating episodes.

2. The diet is a problem if it is "extreme and unhealthy", involving many difficult-to-follow dietary rules that, if adhered to, lead to nutritional deficiencies.

The therapist should emphasize how these two characteristics of dysfunctional dieting cause various problems for the patient. Specifically, it should be highlighted that this type of diet is harmful because of the following reasons:

- It causes concerns about eating, reducing concentration levels in many everyday activities, such as working, watching television, reading a book, or spending time with friends.
- It is emotionally stressful, creating strong concerns about food and potentially causing anxiety and feelings of guilt every time one eats.
- It damages interpersonal relationships because it makes it difficult to eat with others, go out for dinner, or eat food prepared by others.
- It maintains binge-eating episodes (*referring to the patient's personal formulation*). Adopting extreme and rigid dietary rules and the tendency to react extremely and negatively to the almost inevitable breaking of these rules (e.g., consuming a forbidden food or one that triggers a binge-eating episode) leads to a temporary loss of control over eating. This behaviour is followed by a return to an increasingly strict diet to cope with the perceived "failure" of not adhering to the dietary rules. Additionally, binge-eating episodes are further promoted by the biological pressure exerted by severe calorie restriction.

14.2 Identifying Dietary Rules

Once the reasons for addressing unhealthy and rigid eating have been explained to the patient and the patient has agreed that they might warrant addressing, the next step involves identifying the patient's specific dietary rules. It is not always easy to do this because some patients may deny having them or struggle to recognize them as problematic. Clues to dietary rules can, however, be gleaned from the asterisks they write on their monitoring records, and their description of lapses in eating control. The urge to binge can be particularly revealing of the breaking of a dietary rule.

In this module, the patient is encouraged to write, in real time, the dietary rules that they identify in the Comments column of the monitoring record. If it is difficult for them to identify their rules, the therapist might ask the patient questions about whether they would readily eat at a restaurant or at someone else's house, or accept a last-minute invitation to dinner. Dietary rules can vary in content, but generally involve the type and quantity of food, foods to avoid, times when eating is allowed or not allowed, and other rules such as not eating more than others present, not eating unless one has earned it (e.g., not having done enough exercise), and not eating food with unknown calorie content.

14.3 General Strategy for Addressing Dietary Rules

The principles we use to address dietary rules are as follows [2]:

1. *Identifying a specific dietary rule and the reason behind it.* Find the motivation behind a dietary rule by asking the patient about concerns they would have if they were to break it. Dietary rules often have the aim of losing weight or preventing weight gain. In patients with binge-eating episodes, however, the goal might be to avoid breaking a rule that could lead to overeating.
2. *Exploring the likely consequences of breaking the dietary rule.* Emphasize that breaking a dietary rule does not necessarily lead to weight gain or stop weight loss. The consequences depend on the amount of food consumed overall. Additionally, teaching the patient to break the rule by following specific guidelines can prevent the onset of binge-eating episodes.
3. *Devising a plan with the patient.* Collaborate with the patient on a plan to break a dietary rule. The plan should include what, when, where, and with whom the patient will eat, and how they should handle the period following the event. Binge eating should be forestalled at such times by applying the "things to say and do" procedure.
4. *Examining the outcome of breaking the rule.* Explore the outcome, considering the concerns and beliefs about breaking the rule that the patient expressed before doing so, comparing them with what actually happened. Reiterate the potential benefits of freeing oneself from such rules.
5. *Discussing a plan to continue breaking dietary rules systematically.* Encourage the patient to break a rule until it no longer holds significance for them. It is advisable to adopt this procedure for each dietary rule identified.

14.4 Addressing Food Avoidance

One of the most common unhealthy and rigid dietary rules to address is avoiding certain foods, e.g., carbs. This phenomenon, called "food avoidance", typically represents the best type of dietary rule to address first, as it is straightforward in its form and easy to identify. Patients who avoid certain foods often believe that eating them will inevitably lead to weight gain and perhaps even a binge-eating episode. This belief can be debunked by asking the patient to introduce an avoided food into a meal or snack on a day when they feel in control and able to resist the impulse/desire to binge. To do this, the patient needs to plan when and how much of the avoided food they will eat, what they will do if there is any leftover food (e.g., the rest of a chocolate bar), and what they will do afterwards (e.g., engage in a distracting activity). This way, the patient can become aware that a binge-eating episode is not the inevitable consequence of breaking a dietary rule. Repeating this experiment several times leads to no longer perceiving that particular food as dangerous. Moreover, when the feared consequences (i.e., weight gain and binge eating) do not arise, the patient gradually comes to view the dietary rule as a problem rather than a useful means of controlling weight and eating.

Regarding the belief that breaking a rule will lead to weight gain, exposing the patient to some avoided foods, in combination with weekly weighing, can debunk this belief. However, the therapist must emphasize that there are no inherently "fattening" foods: it all depends on the quantities consumed. Repeated consumption of the avoided food and analyzing its implications gradually undermines the patient's perceived need to avoid certain foods, allowing them to become more flexible, and reducing their concerns about eating.

The procedure we use to address food avoidance involves three steps. The first step is to emphasize to the patient that (i) there are no fattening foods (it depends on the quantity: a calorie is a calorie) and that (ii) avoiding foods ruins a person's social life. The second step is to ask the patient to create a list of foods they avoid for fear of gaining weight or having a binge-eating episode. This can be achieved by the patient going to a supermarket or looking at grocery store website to compile a comprehensive list of foods they avoid [2]. The list should then be divided into four groups based on the perceived ease of incorporating them into meals, from the least threatening (Group #1) to the most threatening (Group #4) (see Fig. 14.1). The third step is to gradually encourage the patient to introduce avoided foods, starting with Group #1. On their monitoring record, the patient should plan to introduce the avoided food in one of their daily meals or snacks. When they have successfully introduced it, they should write the word NEW next to the inserted food in real time, and in the Comments column write what they felt before and after eating it. In some cases, the therapist may advise the patient to use the "things to say and do" procedure after introducing the avoided food if they feel the urge to binge.

Dealing with each avoided food would require many sessions, so we also recommend selecting representative foods within the same category, as successfully addressing representative foods typically reduces concern about the entire category. The amount of food consumed does not necessarily have to be large enough to represent a whole portion, even though the ultimate goal is for the patient to be able to eat average amounts of food without difficulty. However, this result may need to be achieved gradually. The systematic introduction of avoided foods should continue until the patient is no longer anxious about eating them.

Here are examples of how the therapist can address some comments from a patient reluctant to tackle food avoidance:

Group 1	*Group 2*	*Group 3*	*Group 4*
Bananas	*Whole-milk yogurt*	*Barley and spelt*	*Potato chips*
Grapes	*Boiled potatoes*	*Tuna in oil*	*Cakes and snacks*
Biscuits	*Whole milk*	*Avocado*	*Cream-based ice cream*
Chickpeas and peas	*Red meat*	*Shortbread cookies*	*Dried fruits*
Non-wholegrain cereals	*Salmon*	*Fresh cheeses*	*Pizza*
	Muesli	*Fruit sorbet*	*Flatbread*
	Eggs		*Aged cheeses*
			Butter

Fig. 14.1 List of avoided foods compiled by a patient

Patient: Eating certain foods goes against a healthy diet.

Therapist: Certainly, what you're saying is valid, and the goal of our work is not to have an unhealthy diet. Instead, it's about enabling you to freely choose what to eat without being influenced by fears and concerns.

Patient: But how do I know how much of that food I should eat?

Therapist: At this moment, the point is for you to try to face the fears you have about that food. If eating even a small amount scares you, having a couple of mouthfuls is okay. We'll work on eating a full portion later on.

Patient: I just don't like some foods.

Therapist: I understand, but I want you to think about whether you genuinely dislike one food and have never liked it or if, in reality, you fear that it might have consequences for your body. If you genuinely don't like it, you can choose not to include it. However, it's important that you try to eat some to prevent your concerns about that food from persisting. Sometimes it's worth experimenting and trying a food you don't like (everyone does it occasionally) to get to the bottom of your reaction.

Patient: Some foods can be skipped, like fruit juices; why do I have to include them?

Therapist: You're right; there are some things that you may choose not to eat or drink at all as they're not essential to your diet. However, remember that what we are focusing on now is you being free to choose what to eat without concerns about the consequences. So, if including that food causes some worry, even if it's an item you'll only include occasionally in the future, on special occasions, it's important that you try to include it. This is to prevent your concerns from persisting and influencing your dietary choices.

By the end of the work on food avoidance, the patient should be able to eat most of the foods on their initial list without feeling guilty or anxious about weight gain, or afraid they will provoke a binge-eating episode.

14.5 Addressing Other Dietary Rules

Dysfunctional dieting involves specific dietary rules on not only what to eat, but also when, where, and how. These should be addressed via a similar approach to that above, homing in on the belief that is maintaining the dietary rule, practicing breaking it, and evaluating the implications. The therapist should always emphasize the positive aspects of breaking dietary rules. The following paragraphs describe some specific rules that may need to be addressed [2].

Dietary rules regarding when to eat. These dietary rules were already addressed in Step One, which introduced the regular eating procedure. If, however, the patient is still encountering difficulties in regulating meal frequency, they do need to be broken down. The therapist needs to remind the patient that there is no right or wrong time to eat, no differences in nutrient absorption based on the time of day, and delaying eating as much as possible makes binge-eating episodes more likely. Eating regularly at intervals of no more than 4 hours has several advantages: (i) it provides structure to eating habits (and the day); (ii) it addresses one of the three forms of dieting (skipping meals, the other two being eliminating foods and reducing portions); (iii) it breaks the cycle of binge-eating episodes and dietary restriction; and (iv) it reduces concerns about eating. The therapist should encourage the patient to adopt behaviours that facilitate regular eating, for example, eating at regular intervals (not letting more than 4 hours pass between each food intake), planning mealtimes in advance, and not eating between meals. The patient should be reminded how to use the "things to say and do" procedure if they feel the urge/desire to eat between planned meals.

Dietary rules regarding how much to eat. The therapist should explain to patients that the "right" amount of food to eat overall is that conducive to maintaining a stable, healthy weight. This applies to daily intake, meals, and portion sizes. To attain a reasonable and healthy weight loss, the quantity of food to consume is that necessary to achieve a negative calorie balance of 500 kcal per day, which can be flexibly planned by referring to the guidelines described in Chap. 12.

Dietary rules about not eating in front of others. These rules significantly compromise social functioning and damage relationships. Generally, they stem from the dysfunctional belief that others will notice how much the patient eats and think that they are greedy, or lack willpower or control. The therapist should help the patient understand that the underlying error in their reasoning behind this rule is assuming that others have the same way of thinking about food control as the patient does. In general, other people do not even notice what others are eating, and even if they do, they do not pass judgment their eating behaviour.

Dietary rules about eating less than others present. This dietary rule highlights a thinking error called "generalization": the patient draws general conclusions about how much others eat from a single moment, without considering either what they ate earlier in the day or will eat later, or their energy expenditure, weight, gender or age. Additionally, to convey the nonsensical nature of this rule, the therapist can draw a parallel with breathing, asking the patient if they have ever thought about trying to breathe less than others.

Dietary rules about not eating unless hungry. The therapist should discuss with the patient that there's nothing special about resisting eating and eating only when hungry. Extreme hunger is a condition that alters our thinking and behaviour, often negatively, and can lead to uncontrolled eating behaviours like binge-eating episodes.

Dietary rules about not eating unless earned. The therapist can point out to the patient that our bodies expend energy even when at rest through basal metabolism and diet-induced thermogenesis. Food is a necessity, not a reward.

Dietary rules about avoiding eating out. Eating at restaurants, pizzerias, fast-food joints, and buffets is part of the joy of living, and refusing to do so cannot fail to compromise social life. Rules on not eating out are related to the underlying fear of eating foods of unknown calorie composition and/or eating in front of others. In this case, in addition to following the instructions for these two specific rules, it is advisable to ask the patient to list social eating situations that they avoid and start facing up to them, beginning with those that create the least anxiety.

14.6 Addressing Dysfunctional Reactions to Dietary Rule-Breaking

To effectively tackle dysfunctional reactions stemming from breaking dietary rules, a strategic intervention involving identifying and applying standard cognitive behavioural procedures is indicated. Common instances, arising from dichotomous reasoning patterns, include:

- Breaking a dietary rule is interpreted as evidence of having lost control ("*I've ruined my diet.*") and lack of willpower ("*I've failed.*").
- Breaking a dietary rule has led to the abandonment of control over eating ("*I've lost control; I might as well give up.*").

The therapist should help patients to recognize that control is manifested through adopting *flexible* dietary guidelines rather than adhering strictly to extreme and inflexible rules. It is important that patients with these reactions be helped to detect this kind of "all-or-nothing'" thinking in real time, question what it means, and respond accordingly. With practice, they should get better at not resorting to self-criticism and/or binge eating.

References

1. Cooper Z, Calugi S, Dalle GR. Controlling binge eating and weight: a treatment for binge eating disorder worth researching? Eat Weight Disord. 2019;25(4):1105–9. https://doi.org/10.1007/s40519-019-00734-4.
2. Fairburn CG. Cognitive behavior therapy and eating disorders. New York: Guilford Press; 2008.
3. Dalle Grave R, Calugi S. Cognitive behavior therapy for adolescents with eating disorders. New York: Guilford Press; 2020.

Overvaluation of Shape and Weight Module

15

Abstract

Overvaluation of shape and weight (i.e., judging oneself predominantly or even exclusively in terms of shape and weight) is encountered in over 50% of patients with binge eating disorder (BED). It needs to be addressed by the treatment because it contributes to maintaining binge-eating episodes and predicts a negative treatment outcome in BED patients. This module addresses the overvaluation of shape and weight through a personalized set of specific strategies and procedures that include the creation of the personal formulation of overvaluation of shape and weight and how to address societal pressures, the marginalization of other life domains, shape checking, and shape avoidance.

Overvaluation of shape and weight is a term used to describe a person's self-evaluation based predominantly or even exclusively on shape, weight, and their control [1]. This characteristic is common in patients with anorexia nervosa and bulimia nervosa [2] and, as noted in Chap. 1, is encountered in over 50% of patients with BED [3]. When present, it needs to be addressed because it contributes to maintaining binge-eating episodes (see Chap. 2) and predicts a negative treatment outcome in BED patients [3, 4]. Persistence of overvaluation of shape and weight also predicts relapse in patients with BED who achieve abstinence from binge eating through behavioural treatments [5]. The patient likely has this characteristic if they score ≥4 on one or both questions in Table 4.3 [6].

Addressing overvaluation of shape and weight takes time. Therefore, if present, it is best to start this work early in Step Two. Once the process has begun, it should remain a consistent focus of each session. We discourage patients with this psychopathology from any attempt to lose weight until they reach a persistent remission from their eating disorder, as dieting perpetuates the overvaluation of shape and weight.

R. Dalle Grave et al., *Cognitive Behavior Therapy for Binge Eating Disorder*, https://doi.org/10.1007/978-3-031-71456-6_15

It is important to always bear in mind that addressing overvaluation of shape and weight in patients with BED and clinical obesity (see Sect. 4.3.1 and Table 4.4 for the definition) is a challenge for both the therapist and the patient. The therapist must unconditionally accept the patient, without weight bias or prejudice, if they are to bring about any change and reduce the importance they attribute to shape and weight. It is also crucial for the therapist to truly understand how the patient with clinical obesity experiences their body shape in a culture that associates obesity with greed or laziness, and sends the message that weight loss is just a matter of willpower.

When exploring the patient's overvaluation of shape and weight, it is inevitable that the therapist feels a sense of discomfort and powerlessness while listening to their emotional distress. Patients often report upsetting experiences that have reinforced feelings of discrimination, such as being unable to sit comfortably in a movie theatre or on an aeroplane, having difficulty finding clothes to wear, and/or being criticized by other healthcare professionals for their weight. For these reasons, therapists should be empathetic, demonstrating an understanding of how challenging it is for patients with higher weight to live in our society. Empathy is a necessary skill for validating patients' negative feelings about shape and weight and helping them achieve cognitive change. Recovery will entail a difficult journey from entrenched internalized negative societal prejudices against people with clinical obesity to positive self-acceptance. This will, however, be the key to promoting the behavioural changes necessary for improving self-evaluation without pursuing unrealistic weight-loss goals.

The CBT strategies and procedures for addressing overvaluation of shape and weight adapted for patients with BED are as follows:

- Identifying the overvaluation of shape and weight and its consequences
- Constructing the personalized formulation of overvaluation of shape and weight
- Developing a plan to address the overvaluation of shape and weight
- Addressing societal pressures
- Enhancing the importance of other self-evaluation domains
- Addressing body shape checking (weight checking has already been discussed in Step One)
- Addressing body shape avoidance (weight avoidance has already been discussed in Step One)

15.1 Identifying Overvaluation of Shape and Weight and Its Consequences

Discussing how a patient judges their self-worth is a crucial step for patients with BED. This should be done with the aid of a pie chart to illustrate their self-evaluation schema. In our experience, almost all patients manage to grasp this concept.

The therapist should initiate the discussion by explaining that most people evaluate themselves based on the success they achieve in areas of life they deem important. Common domains of self-evaluation include relationships with family and friends, and achievements at work, sports, and other activities. The therapist should provide examples, explaining that a person may judge themself based on their work achievements, feeling good when they reach their goals but feeling bad when they do not. They may also judge themselves on the quality of their relationships, feeling happy when receiving positive recognition from peers, being appreciated for their actions, and actively participating in activities, but feeling sad and frustrated when facing criticism or perceiving disinterest from others. Generally, individuals have multiple areas of self-evaluation, and not all areas are given the same importance. However, it is essential to emphasize the need to distinguish between what is generally important in life and what represents a specific self-evaluation domain for the individual. If a person feels very negatively and for an extended period of time when a certain aspect of their life is not going well, it is likely an important self-evaluation domain for them. For instance, if a person judges themselves based on their work achievements, they may develop an intensely negative and enduring emotional reaction when they fail to meet their own expectations. If the failure persists, it can lead to a negative self-evaluation.

Once the therapist ensures that the patient understands this concept, they encourage them to draw up a written list of what they consider important life domains, and how they evaluate themselves in these areas. At this stage, the patient may omit weight and body shape from the list, and, if so, the therapist must address this topic, as in the following excerpt from a conversation between a therapist and a patient:

Therapist: You've listed friendships, work, family and your romantic relationship. Does anything seem to be missing, or do these appear to be the important areas in your life that you use to value yourself?

Patient: Yes, those are all of them. I've thought about it and can't think of anything else.

Therapist: Let's try to reflect on it together, perhaps by considering why you're here and our work together. What prompted you to start therapy?

Patient: (*pauses, a bit puzzled*) I have no control over my eating, and I am too conditioned by my shape and weight.

Therapist: Exactly. Why are you so conditioned by your shape and weight?

Patient: Because I am overweight and... because my shape and weight are so important to me, I guess. They have become more important than other things that used to matter.

Therapist: Exactly! So, based on what you're saying, I think we'll need to add something to the list you wrote.

Patient: Yes, you're right, weight and shape. I don't know why I didn't think of it before. I took it for granted; that's the most important of all... I am too big.

Therapist: Okay. Let's add "weight and shape" to the list.

Once the list is complete, to assess the relative importance the patient attributes to each domain, the therapist should enquire specifically about the intensity and duration of the adverse reaction when things go wrong in that particular area [7]. The more intense and enduring the negative reaction, the larger the corresponding slice in the pie chart should be. This analysis allows for the creation of a provisional self-evaluation pie chart in which each slice reflects the importance that the patient assigns to each area of their life. Typically, a patient with BED and overvaluation of shape and weight has a pie chart with a few slices (few self-evaluation domains) and a predominant slice (that of shape and weight), as illustrated in Fig. 15.1. Most patients recognize themselves in their pie chart and spontaneously acknowledge that they give too much importance to their shape and weight.

As a homework assignment, the patient should be encouraged to review their pie chart daily for a week and reflect on whether it accurately represents their attitudes and behaviours [7]. To do this, the patient can draw their pie chart on the back of the monitoring record at the end of each day. In the next session, the pie chart should be revisited, and the size of the slices revaluated. Since it is almost inevitable that the patient, as in the transcript above, attributes overvaluation of shape and weight to being overweight, it is important to explain the difference between overvaluation of shape and weight and physical appearance to the patient. The therapist should tactfully inform them that there are individuals with normal weight and even underweight, according to the BMI cut-offs, who overvalue shape and weight. Furthermore, many people with clinical obesity (about 80%) [8] do not judge themselves predominantly on their shape and weight, even if they are dissatisfied with their bodies. In most people, body dissatisfaction does not have a negative impact on their self-evaluation or their abilities in relational contexts. Generally, most patients grasp this concept, and some admit to admiring individuals who can accept or even appreciate their bodies, even if they have a BMI in the obesity range.

The therapist's next task will be to assist the patient in assessing the implications of having a pie chart with one predominant slice and few others. The therapist might say something like: "*In the short term, it may be advantageous to judge oneself in only one area (e.g., shape and weight) as compared to several areas (e.g., academic performance, relationships, interests, sports and work achievements, personal*

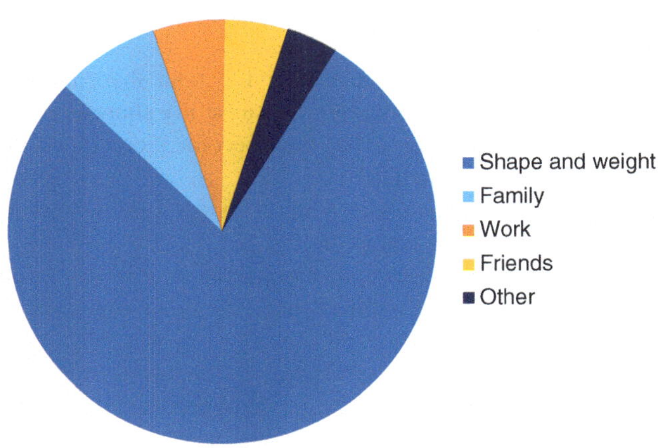

Fig. 15.1 Pie chart representing the self-evaluation system of a patient with BED and overvaluation of shape and of weight

qualities, etc.) that are more difficult to control, but in the medium to long term, this leads to various negative consequences." Then, the therapist should explain the negative consequences of evaluating oneself in one predominant area, namely:

- *It is at high risk of failure*. Using the pie chart as a reference, the therapist should reflect with the patient that when something goes wrong in their control of shape and weight, as this is the principal domain, this will inevitably lead to the whole self-evaluation system collapsing. The end result is that patients judge themselves negatively overall, as the other domains are too small to make up for perceived failure in this one.
- *It is problematic*. Maintaining a good self-evaluation mainly through the control of shape and weight is problematic for three reasons:
  - Shape and weight are not entirely under the control of will: they are largely influenced by genetics. One can manipulate them in the short term, but to do so on a long-term basis requires considerable and sustained effort, and one pays a price as a result. It is mainly something one just has to accept.
  - There will always be other people who seem more attractive.
  - Judging oneself in this way leads to doing harmful things that maintain the eating disorder, such as adopting dysfunctional diets, engaging in frequent body checking behaviours, and/or avoiding exposing the body.
- *It restricts life and is self-perpetuating*. The exclusive focus on shape and weight marginalizes other areas of life, reducing the individual's interests to the body alone. The therapist should emphasize how this inevitably limits commitment to the other important areas of life (e.g., relationships, work, hobbies) that generally contribute to developing a functional, stable, and articulated self-assessment system.

Attempting to exemplify these aspects, the therapist can ask the patient, adopting both short and long-term perspectives, to assess the consequences of having a predominant focus. At the end of this discussion, the therapist should ask the patient to weigh up the pros and cons of directly addressing their overvaluation of shape and weight. In our clinical experience, most patients agree to address this issue as part of the treatment because they report that the importance they give to their body is one of the main reasons that prompted them to seek help.

The pie chart is a tool that the therapist can use again towards the end of the therapeutic process, having the patient redraw it and assess their progress in terms of psychopathological change.

15.2 Creating the Personal Formulation of Overvaluation of Shape and Weight

After agreeing with the patient that shape and weight are their most important domains of self-evaluation, the next step is to collaboratively build the personal formulation of overvaluation of shape and weight and with the patient. To achieve this, the therapist first educates the patient on the main mechanisms that maintain the overvaluation evaluation and then helps them identify those that seem to be at play in their case (see Fig. 15.2).

- *General and individual social pressures*. The therapist should explain that "general" and "individual" social pressures can contribute to the development of a self-evaluation based on weight and body shape and its maintenance. General social pressures are those that lead a person to want to conform to the widespread societal standard of beauty based on thinness. Patients with BED live in a society that fuels concerns about the body, as it exalts thinness and fosters negative judgments about individuals with clinical obesity. Additionally, some patients are exposed to specific individual social pressures—in the family or at work, for example—that amplify the effect of general pressures in contributing to maintaining a negative body image.
- *Marginalization of other areas of life*. Having an overvaluation of shape and weight inevitably reduces the importance attributed to other areas of life that could help diminish the significance of shape and weight in self-evaluation.
- *Body checking*. This behavioural expression of body concern is manifested by a subgroup of patients with BED. It involves frequent checking of body shape and weight, usually by pinching, weighing, looking in the mirror, and comparing one's body to others. In some cases, body checking can have a positive short-term effect, reassuring the individual that their body weight and shape have not changed. However, in the long term, it has a negative impact, contributing to maintaining the overvaluation of shape and weight through the mechanisms described in Table 15.1.
- *Body avoidance*. This is a typical behavioural expression of body concern, and is very common among patients with BED and clinical obesity. It refers to avoiding situations (the beach, clothes shops, exercise classes, etc.) in which patients think that they would feel very uncomfortable about their body shape [9]. Body avoidance has a positive short-term effect by reducing the distress associated with body exposure. Still, in the long term, it contributes to maintaining the overvaluation of shape and weight through the mechanisms described in Table 15.1.

The next step is to develop a personalized action plan that should focus on the main maintenance processes identified in the patient's personal formulation of

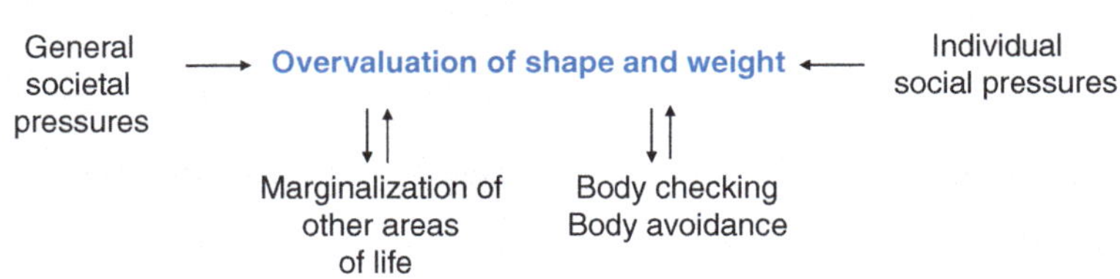

Fig. 15.2 Main maintenance mechanisms of overvaluation of shape and weight in a patient with BED and higher weight

Table 15.1 Mechanisms through which body checking and body avoidance maintain the overvaluation of shape and weight

• Frequently checking, touching, and measuring the body fuels body shape concerns (they are never far from your mind).
• Focusing on disliked body parts amplifies perceived flaws (you only see the parts you don't like).
• Superficial observation of the bodies of atypical individuals (e.g., models or actors), a subgroup of thin people, or those with "special" features (e.g., a flat stomach) only intensifies the mistaken perception that one's own body has the wrong shape.
Body Avoidance
• It prevents having a clear idea of how one appears (like an ostrich with its head in the sand).
• It does not help overcome anxiety associated with occasions when the body is exposed (e.g., swimming, exercising in public).
• It becomes entirely dependent on a person's fear of how they appear to themselves and others, and consequently, these negative predictions and fears are never tested.
• It acts as a barrier to functional socialization, intimacy with a partner, and daily activities such as buying new clothes or going out with friends

overvaluation of shape and weight. In most cases, three complementary strategies are used to address: (i) societal pressures, (ii) the marginalization of other life areas, and (iii) expressions of overvaluation (i.e., body checking and body avoidance).

15.3 Addressing Social Pressures

Unfortunately, there is little that can be done to reduce the general societal pressure to be thin that patients with BED and clinical obesity suffer, and it is often challenging to tackle the individual social pressures they experience. However, the therapist should help the patient become aware of these societal pressures and their negative impact on individuals with clinical obesity. It is also important to help the patient understand that negative societal attitudes towards people with clinical obesity are unjustified—simply the result of bias and ignorance—as various studies indicate that individual body weight is the result of a complex interaction between genetic and environmental risk factors. The patient should be encouraged to ask themselves, "*Is it my problem or a problem of society in general?*" [9]

If the patient agrees that it is society's problem, they should be encouraged to distance themselves from these biases and avoid being negatively influenced. It is also helpful to discuss possible strategies for coping with societal pressures with the patient. These can be simple, such as ignoring them and responding to criticism assertively, or more active, such as writing a letter to a newspaper and/or joining a group that fights prejudice against people with clinical obesity.

If the patient is experiencing social pressure within their own family, the therapist should assess whether involving other significant individuals in the treatment would be helpful. This could enable the most critical individuals to be educated, discussing with them and the patient how they might modulate their critical attitudes toward the patient's eating, body shape and weight.

N.B. Patients with internalized weight stigma should be helped using the strategies and procedures described in Chap. 17.

15.4 Addressing the Marginalization of Other Life Domains

To enhance the importance of other areas of self-evaluation, the following steps should be employed (when discussing each step, the therapist should play an active, proactive and encouraging role, emphasizing their significance and motivate the patient for change) [2]:

- *Explain the rationale for the intervention.* The first step is, as always, to educate the patient on why they need to address the marginalization of other life domains, clarifying that increasing their importance or adding to them will help break the dominance of shape and weight, providing opportunities for other life experiences that are not only fun, but can help to reduce their preoccupation with shape and weight indirectly.
- *Identify new activities.* The patient should reflect on interests they had before developing clinical obesity and/or BED (e.g., sports, hobbies) or consider activities they would like to try that they have never done before, perhaps those practiced by their peers. At this stage, it is crucial to explore all possibilities to provide the patient with ample choices. Then, the pros and cons of engaging in each identified domain must be assessed.
- *Select one or two domains to work on.* It is preferable to suggest that patients choose areas involving other people because they are more likely to be sustained over time and contribute to developing a positive self-evaluation.
- *Ensure patient engagement in identified domains.* The therapist should ask the patient to report their activity in the monitoring record's Comments column, and discuss any obstacles they encountered. The proactive problem-solving procedure described in Chap. 13 could be helpful at this point in finding suitable solutions for difficulties encountered in engaging in new areas of life. Patient should be encouraged to work on enhancing the chosen domain(s) most days of the week.
- *Review progress weekly.* Once this procedure has been introduced, it should be a regular item on the agenda. The therapist should encourage the patient to consistently implement established activities, engage in new activities, and help overcome encountered difficulties. Towards the end of the programme, the patient should be asked to redraw their pie chart. If the work has been effective, the patient will notice that they have increased the number and/or size of the other slices and decreased the size attributed to weight and body shape.

Interests typically developed during this programme include reconnecting with friends, resuming a hobby or, in some cases, practicing a sport. Often, this procedure yields additional benefits, such as building new relationships and increasing self-confidence.

15.5 Addressing Shape Checking

Shape checking is a potent maintenance mechanism of overvaluation of shape and weight, and should be addressed first in most cases. This behaviour usually aims to monitor body shape and/or check if it has changed. Shape checking is common among people without eating issues, but it manifests more frequently and in unusual ways in those with overvaluation of shape and weight [1, 7]. Typical shape checking in patients with BED include the following:

- Visual checking (e.g., often inspecting specific body parts in the mirror or any reflective surface with a hypercritical attitude)
- Measurement checking (e.g., measuring body circumferences such as waist, hips, thighs, and/or wrists)
- Tactile checking (e.g., pinching fat folds to measure their size, wearing tight clothes to see how they fit)
- Comparison checking (e.g., looking at thinner people or specific features of others, such as a flat stomach or slim, long or muscular legs, scrutinizing social media and media models or actors, being interested in the weight and body sizes of others)
- Reassurance checking (e.g., seeking reassurance from others about one's body shape).

The first step in addressing these behaviours is to describe to the patient the main forms of shape checking, and how these maintain and intensify the overvaluation of shape and weight (see Table 15.1). The second step is to explain to the patient that people are often unaware that they are doing these things, and that they should monitor the shape checking behaviours they catch themselves doing over the course of 2 days in the last column of their monitoring record. This will allow them to assess the frequency of episodes and explore the thoughts and emotions associated with them.

The third step is to review with the patient the motivation behind the shape checking behaviour that they have become aware of and its consequences. The following questions may be helpful in this regard [7]:

- Why did you check your body shape?
- Why did you check your body shape so frequently?
- Which part of your body did you look at?
- How did you feel after body checking?
- What effects do you think body checking has on you?

This should lead to the conclusion that shape checking increases body dissatisfaction.

The fourth step is to discuss with the patient which dysfunctional shape checking behaviours to interrupt (e.g., measuring the sizes of various body circumferences, checking for space between thighs, pinching skin folds, looking at the stomach when sitting, wearing tight clothes) and which ones to modify (e.g., use of mirrors, comparison checking).

To interrupt a dysfunctional checking behaviour, it is first necessary for the patient to become aware of it in real time by writing it in the last column of the monitoring record, along with their reason for doing it. This should make it easier for the patient to understand what they are trying to achieve through this behaviour, and to learn to interrupt "cold turkey". As with weight checking (addressed in Step One), concern about body shape may transiently increase but diminish as the patient gains control of this behaviour. However, if a patient finds it difficult to interrupt shape checking, they should be encouraged to identify triggering situations (e.g., after eating, when undressing) and devise and implement strategies to resist the urge (e.g., not undressing in front of a mirror, or doing something manual instead of pinching fat folds).

Regarding behaviours to be modified, the goal is to reduce their frequency and change their nature to achieve functional control of body shape. To this end, the therapist should always discuss the appropriate use of mirrors, particularly the purpose of looking in the mirror, as well as the normal frequency and time spent doing so. The patient should be educated that there are no healthy or useful reasons to look in the mirror, other than to check their hair and clothes in the morning after dressing or before going out.

For patients reporting frequent comparison checking, the therapist should suggest that this can be overcome by addressing the two typical biases associated with this behaviour [7]:

1. *Subject bias* (e.g., comparing oneself to someone young and attractive)
2. *Evaluation bias* (i.e., looking at other people's bodies superficially and non-judgementally but being hypercritical and strict towards one's own body).

The patient should be encouraged to reduce the frequency of such comparisons, become aware of the two biases in real time, broaden their attentional focus (e.g., looking at hair and shoes), and observe other characteristics of the person (e.g., personality). This is also helpful in prompting the patient to become aware of body diversity. In cases in which the comparison is focused on social media, celebrities in magazines or other media, a useful strategy might be to inform the patient that such images do not represent realistic body models, as most, if not all, have been retouched (there are numerous examples of the "Photoshop effect" on the internet that could help them understand this).

15.6 Addressing Shape Avoidance

Shape avoidance is another typical expression of overvaluation of shape and weight, and is common in patients with clinical obesity [10]. Avoiding situations that may cause discomfort due to the need to expose body shape maintains body dissatisfaction and overvaluation of shape and weight through the mechanisms described in

Table 15.1. Typical body avoidance behaviours include (i) avoiding looking at one's body, (ii) avoiding touching one's body, and (iii) avoiding exposing one's body to others.

The first step in addressing body avoidance is to illustrate this process to the patient, drawing on some of their experiences and explaining how they act to reinforce body dissatisfaction. The therapist should help the patient conclude that it is better to face up to situations that they would prefer to avoid if only to test their predictions and the negative consequences they fear [9].

The second step is to help patients plan specific behavioural tasks that they can use to overcome their fears. The plan should involve the progressive exposure of specific body parts, starting with those that cause less discomfort (e.g., going out with three-quarter-length sleeves rather than long sleeves). The patient should also be encouraged to anticipate the consequences of body shape exposure, write their predictions on their monitoring record and, with the therapist's assistance, plan how to achieve the goal and face the anticipated negative consequences [9].

The third step is to inquire about how the attempt went, and whether the feared negative consequences occurred. The therapist should emphasize the positive aspects of the outcome, including the fact that the patient overcame their reluctance to try it, and reevaluate with the patient what they have learned from the experience. This way, the patient is assisted in gradually getting used to the sight and feel of their own body, and ultimately feel comfortable exposing it in the presence of others. Usually, this process does not require many sessions, and significantly reduces dysfunctional body avoidance, conferring secondary benefits such as increased socialization opportunities.

15.6.1 Intervention Outcomes

The CBT strategies and related complementary procedures used to address overvaluation of shape and weight gradually erode its main expressions (i.e., shape checking and shape avoidance), improving the importance of other life domains and better managing social and societal pressures. This progressively reduces the patient's body concerns and the significance they attribute to shape and weight in their self-evaluation system. This process may also be consolidated by addressing internalized weight stigma in those who present this feature (see Chap. 17).

Vignette

The patient is a 23-year-old young woman who began experiencing recurrent binge-eating episodes without compensatory behaviours at the age of 19 after losing about 15 kg (from 72 kg to 57 kg) by following a low-carbohydrate diet prescribed by a nutritionist. In the following years, she alternated prolonged periods characterized by recurrent binge-eating episodes and dysregulated eating and overeating with others in which she followed a dysfunctional diet, rapidly losing weight (5–6 kg in a month), which she then regained with the recurrence of binge-eating episodes. These behaviours resulted in a progressive weight gain, up to 85 kg, and the development of overvaluation of shape and weight. The patient reported being very unhappy and dissatisfied with her weight and body shape, feeling embarrassed about her weight, especially when meeting new people. She also reported avoiding going to the pool and practicing her previous hobbies, like Latin American dancing, because she believed others would ridicule her. The patient took little care of her physical appearance, did not wear makeup, wore loose, dark clothes, and avoided weighing herself. Overvaluation of shape and weight also led her to eschew social situations, such as going out to dinner with friends, and intermittently adopt strict diets, which were inevitably interrupted by binge-eating episodes. Additionally, with every gain in weight, she experienced a strong negative reaction that lasted for days, during which she would not leave the house.

In Step Two, after agreeing with the therapist to postpone any weight-loss attempts, she began addressing the marginalization of life domains by enrolling in a Latin American dance class, because dancing had always been her passion. To her surprise, she was welcomed warmly by the teacher and other members of the school. Attending the dance class allowed her to meet friendly people and spend enjoyable moments with them after lessons. She started taking better care of her physical appearance, and buying new makeup and colourful clothes. She also began accepting dinner invitations and attending parties her dance classmates had organized.

In addition to the success of the attempt to increase the importance of other self-evaluation domains, the patient ceased dysfunctional shape checking behaviours, such as critically observing her body in the mirror (especially her legs and hips) and comparing herself to thinner women. Dancing helped her become more confident and expose herself to previously avoided situations, such as going to the pool. At the end of Step Two, although the patient was still dissatisfied with her body shape, she realized that her quality of life and self-evaluation had improved thanks to her discontinuing binge-eating episodes and her body image improving, even though she had not lost weight.

References

1. Dalle Grave R, Calugi S. Transdiagnostic cognitive behavioural theory and treatment of body image disturbance in eating disorders: a guide to assessment, treatment, and prevention. In: Cuzzolaro M, Fassino S, editors. Body Image, Eating, and Weight. Cham: Springer; 2018. p. 309–21.
2. Fairburn CG, Cooper Z, Shafran R. Cognitive behaviour therapy for eating disorders: a "transdiagnostic" theory and treatment. Behav Res Ther. 2003;41(5):509–28. https://doi.org/10.1016/s0005-7967(02)00088-8.

3. Grilo CM, White MA, Gueorguieva R, Wilson GT, Masheb RM. Predictive significance of the overvaluation of shape/weight in obese patients with binge eating disorder: findings from a randomized controlled trial with 12-month follow-up. Psychol Med. 2013;43(6):1335–44. https://doi.org/10.1017/s0033291712002097.
4. Masheb RM, Grilo CM. Prognostic significance of two sub-categorization methods for the treatment of binge eating disorder: negative affect and overvaluation predict, but do not moderate, specific outcomes. Behav Res Ther. 2008;46(4):428–37. https://doi.org/10.1016/j.brat.2008.01.004.
5. Grilo CM, Ivezaj V, Gueorguieva R. Overvaluation of shape/weight at posttreatment predicts relapse at 12-month follow-up after successful behaviorally-based treatment of binge-eating disorder. Int J Eat Disord. 2024; https://doi.org/10.1002/eat.24141.
6. Fairburn C, Cooper Z. The Eating Disorder Examination. In: Fairburn C, Wilson G, editors. Binge eating: Nature, assessment, and treatment. Guilford Press: New York; 1993. p. 317–60.
7. Fairburn CG. Cognitive behavior therapy and eating disorders. New York: Guilford Press; 2008.
8. Dalle Grave R, Misconel A, Fasoli D, Calugi S. Overvaluation of shape and weight and associated features in patients without eating disorders seeking treatment for obesity. Obesity. 2020;28(4):733–9. https://doi.org/10.1002/oby.22750.
9. Cooper Z, Fairburn CG, Hawker DM. Cognitive-behavioral treatment of obesity: a clinician's guide. Guilford Press; 2003.
10. Dalle Grave R, Sartirana M, El Ghoch M, Calugi S. Module 5: Addressing weight-loss dissatisfaction. Treating obesity with personalized cognitive behavioral therapy. Cham: Springer; 2018. p. 117–42.

Unrealistic Weight Goals Module 16

Abstract

Satisfaction with the amount of weight lost is one the most critical factors involved in long-term body-weight maintenance. Moreover, a decline in weight-loss satisfaction about 4 to 5 months after starting the treatment is associated with poor long-term weight-loss outcomes. To address these obstacles to weight maintenance, cognitive behavior therapy (CBT) for binge-eating disorder (BED) includes the Unrealistic Weight Goals module, designed to help patients who report "unsatisfactory" weight loss 4–5 months from the start of treatment to arrive at the beginning of the weight-maintenance phase in Step Three satisfied with the weight they have reached. Patients who report a decline in weight-loss satisfaction, assessed session by session via the Weight-Loss Obstacles Questionnaire, are helped to identify the reasons behind their weight-loss dissatisfaction. These reasons generally fall into two main, often interrelated, categories: unrealistic weight-loss expectations and/or dysfunctional primary reasons for weight loss. The goal is to encourage the patient to achieve positive acceptance of their body shape and the weight they have reached with the treatment, balancing change and acceptance—changing what can be changed (lifestyle) and accepting what cannot (i.e., achieving an "ideal" body shape and weight).

The importance we place on addressing unrealistic weight goals is derived from our research findings. Evidence suggests that a crucial cognitive factor involved in weight maintenance is the patient's satisfaction with weight loss [1, 2]. Furthermore, we have observed that a decline in satisfaction with weight loss 4–5 months into the programme—specifically, a score equal to or less than seven on the "satisfaction with weight" item on the Weight-Loss Obstacles Questionnaire (Appendix 4)—can help identify patients who will not be able to maintain the lost weight [3]. Discussing these findings, we hypothesized that dissatisfaction with the results achieved in the weight-loss phase of treatment could cause a decrease in patient motivation and

R. Dalle Grave et al., *Cognitive Behavior Therapy for Binge Eating Disorder*, https://doi.org/10.1007/978-3-031-71456-6_16

reduce adherence to the lifestyle modification necessary for long-term weight maintenance.

In our clinical experience, we usually observe a decrease in satisfaction with the weight loss in patients with unrealistic weight goals and other deferred life goals that they hope to achieve by losing weight (referred to as "primary goals"). For this reason, the Unrealistic Weight Goals module has been designed with the aim of helping the subgroup of patients who express dissatisfaction with weight loss 4–5 months into treatment. The goal is to help them reach the beginning of the weight maintenance phase satisfied with and positively accepting the weight they have lost, laying firm foundations for the right mindset for long-term weight maintenance.

16.1 Identifying Dissatisfaction with Weight Loss and General Strategies for Addressing It

The degree of satisfaction with the weight lost during the Healthy Weight Loss module is assessed by the therapist, session by session, taking into consideration the patient's response to item 15 on the Weight-Loss Obstacles Questionnaire (Appendix 4). This item asks the patient to express their satisfaction with their weight loss on a Likert scale (0–10). If the patient assigns a score of 7 or less to this item, the issue of weight-loss dissatisfaction should be included in the session agenda.

CBT for BED addresses dissatisfaction with weight loss through two different general strategies. If dissatisfaction arises in the first 12 weeks of the Healthy Weight Loss module and is associated with a lower amount of weight loss than the treatment's weekly goal (i.e., 0.5 kg/week), it is addressed through the strategies and procedures described in Chap. 12. This aims to help the patient improve physical activity and eating plan adherence. It is crucial to promptly address early dissatisfaction with weight loss, as it is often associated with dropout [4, 5]. However, if dissatisfaction with weight loss occurs after week 12, it should be addressed using the specific strategies and procedures described in the following paragraphs. Indeed, dissatisfaction with the results achieved in this late phase is likely due to unrealistic weight-loss goals and dysfunctional, unrealistic primary goals rather than obstacles to weight loss, which should have already been largely overcome.

16.2 Identifying Unrealistic Weight Goals and Primary Goals

It is essential to identify why a patient reports being dissatisfied with the amount of weight they have lost. To do this, the therapist can ask something like: "*I noticed that on the Weight-Loss Obstacles Questionnaire, you reported a score lower than seven on the question relating to satisfaction with the weight loss. Is there any specific reason you are dissatisfied with your weight loss?*" Commonly, the patient initially reports generic reasons, such as wanting to lose more weight and/or thinking they would have lost more by this stage. However, if the therapist investigates these feelings in more detail, it usually emerges that the reasons behind the dissatisfaction fall into one or both of the following general categories [6–8]:

1. Unrealistic weight goals
2. Dysfunctional primary goals

Identifying unrealistic weight goals and dysfunctional primary goals can be facilitated by asking the patient to complete the Weight Goals and Primary Goals Questionnaire (see Appendix 5) [7]. The questionnaire has three sections, with the first asking the patient to indicate the following three weight goals:

1. Dream weight: the weight they would ideally like to have (even if it may be unrealistic and unattainable)
2. Desired weight: the weight they want to reach and believe they can achieve
3. Acceptable weight: the highest weight they think they could accept

For each weight goal mentioned above, the patient must report a number in kilograms (or pounds). Sometimes, patients may not have a specific weight goal but want to reach a desired clothing size or lose as much weight as possible. Even if this is the case, they should be encouraged to quantify the desired sizes with a precise number in kilograms (or pounds).

The second section of the Weight Goals and Primary Goals Questionnaire includes specific items on the desired weight, which can be considered the "true" weight-loss goal. The patient is also asked to report why they have indicated that particular desired weight, whether it has changed, and why this change has occurred (if applicable). Another item in this section asks the patient to consider the difficulty they anticipate in reaching and maintaining the desired weight, and how long they have managed to do so in the past.

Finally, the third section of the questionnaire includes questions about primary goals, what the patient expects to achieve by losing weight, and whether this necessarily involves weight loss.

16.3 Addressing Unrealistic Weight Goals

The first step in addressing unrealistic weight goals is to educate the patient on weight regulation and the outcomes typically achieved through weight-loss treatments based on lifestyle modification. The key points to discuss are as follows [9]:

- Weight is partially controlled by genetics and therefore a person can only modify it to a certain extent (e.g., 5–10%) without resorting to weight-loss drugs or bariatric surgery.
- Even individuals who lose a significant amount of weight struggle to maintain it in the long term.

- Without specific weight-maintenance strategies, most people regain one-third of the lost weight after 1 year and the entire lost weight after 5 years.
- Most individuals starting a weight-loss treatment aim to lose more than 5–10% of their weight, and this unrealistic expectation may lead them to abandon the programme or not commit to maintaining the lost weight because they perceive the achieved result as unsatisfactory.
- A 5–10% weight loss has many health benefits and can positively impact quality of life, in addition to reducing major medical complications associated with clinical obesity (see Sect. 4.3.1 and Table 4.4 for the definition).
- A good treatment helps a person change what can be changed and accept what cannot. Striking a balance between change and acceptance is a common goal in medicine, especially in chronic medical conditions such as diabetes mellitus.

Based on this information, the patient should be encouraged to discuss and consider the following three points [9, 10]:

1. Some changes (e.g., 5–10% weight loss) are possible and, while perhaps not ideal, can bring significant benefits.
2. Treatment can successfully address other primary goals associated with personal weight goals, improving quality of life. However, successful outcomes depend on accepting what cannot be changed (acceptance as self-affirmation).
3. Without acceptance of what cannot be changed, there is a high risk of relapse. This is because there is a tendency to underestimate what has been achieved during treatment and to reduce commitment to maintaining the lost weight, as that would be considered pointless.

The second step is to help the patient accept and be satisfied with the weight achieved in the weight-loss phase. To this end, their desired weight goal should be explored, addressing the following topics [9, 10]:

- *Origin of the desired weight.* The therapist should enquire about how the patient arrived at selecting their desired weight. Common responses include medical recommendations, ideal weight charts, a desire to return to a previous lower weight, or the belief that a specific weight is necessary to achieve certain primary goals.
- *Variability of the desired weight.* The therapist should explore whether their desired weight has changed over the years. If so, the reasons behind the change should be discussed.
- *Previous weight-loss attempts.* The patient should be asked if they have been able to reach the desired weight through previous weight-loss attempts. If not, what obstacles did they encounter? If so, why were they unable to maintain that weight?

- *Difficulties and risks in pursuing the desired weight.* The patient should be guided to reflect on the challenges of achieving the desired weight, and whether there are risks associated.
- *Consequences of achieving or not achieving the desired weight.* The therapist should enquire about the patient's realistic expectations regarding whether they will reach the desired weight. How will they interpret this outcome? What actions will they take? Will their life truly change?

The third step is to examine the causes of past failures in maintaining lost weight (if the patient reported them). The therapist should assist in analyzing the phases of weight loss and weight maintenance in previous weight-loss attempts as follows:

- *Weight-loss phase.* Enquire about the patient's initial weight, the duration of the weight-loss phase, the amount lost, and whether or not they achieved their desired weight. Encourage the patient to draw conclusions from their previous experience.
- *Weight-maintenance phase.* Ask the patient if they intentionally decided to start weight maintenance. If so, why? If not, why not? Enquire about the duration of weight maintenance and factors influencing subsequent weight regain. The therapist should prompt the patient to consider three main processes [10]:
  - Unrealistic weight-loss goals and dissatisfaction with achieved weight leading to a lack of commitment to weight maintenance
  - Not knowing how to maintain weight
  - Difficulty adhering to an overly restrictive diet for an extended period

The fourth step is helping the patient assess the benefits of modest weight loss, and the positive changes already achieved through treatment. Encourage the patient to consider improvements in the following areas [9]:

- Physical appearance and clothing size reduction
- General well-being
- Self-confidence
- Medical complications related to clinical obesity (the therapist may suggest repeating blood tests conducted before the weight-loss phase to assess objective improvements)
- Physical fitness (e.g., climbing stairs with less effort, feeling more agile, easily tying shoelaces)

The fifth step is to encourage the patient to write down the pros and cons of continuing to pursue the desired weight, considering the potential advantages, disadvantages, and risks.

Vignette

The patient, a 51-year-old woman with BED and clinical obesity, began the treatment at a weight of 98 kg. She was also suffering from type 2 diabetes and hypertension, which were being managed through medications. After 5 months of treatment, she reached a weight of 86 kg, but her personal goal was 67 kg, a weight she been at the age of 20. After instructing the patient on weight regulation, the therapist asked her to reassess her desired weight by reviewing past weight-loss attempts (she had never been able to return to 67 kg). Underscoring the achievement of a 12 kg weight reduction, the therapist asked the patient to identify any perceived benefits of her current weight. Without hesitation, the patient mentioned several physical benefits. Specifically, she needed less medication to control her blood sugar and blood pressure. She felt more agile, and was capable of walking several kilometres without getting out of breath. Moreover, her self-confidence had improved because she could eat regularly and healthily without bingeing. However, she remained dissatisfied with the weight loss she had achieved, and the fact that her weight had remained stable over the past 3 weeks. She was determined to intensify dietary restriction to reach her desired weight of 67 kg. Hence, the therapist assigned her the task of compiling a list of pros and cons of achieving her desired weight. In the next session, a review of this list revealed that the patient had listed only advantages and no disadvantages to reaching her desired weight. Here follows the dialogue between therapist and patient that ensued:

Therapist: I'm glad you filled out the "pros and cons" table. Did this task help you?

Patient: I guess… However, I could only find advantages to losing more weight.

Therapist: I see (*pointing to the table's pros*). You wrote that if you reached your desired weight, you would have a wider choice of clothes, and be able to play tennis with your friend.

Patient: I'd like to wear a medium size... that would be a good goal. And I'd like to play tennis with my friend.

Therapist: Okay, I understand. I see that your satisfaction score for weight loss is currently 5. Patient: Yes, it is! I think if I manage to reach 67 kg, it would be a ten.

Therapist: Let's consider why you didn't write any disadvantages to reaching your desired weight; what do you think you should do to achieve your goal of 67 kg?

Patient: I don't understand. I'll do the same as I'm already doing!

Therapist: Are you sure? In the last three weeks, your weight has remained stable.

Patient: True (*thoughtful*).

Therapist:	This is a common occurrence. Weight loss tends to plateau after 5–6 months. This is because the lost weight results in a progressive decrease in energy expenditure.
Patient:	Ah... So, if I understand correctly, I need to eat less or exercise more if I want to keep losing weight.
Therapist:	Yes, that's correct. However, before deciding whether to increase calorie restriction or energy expenditure, I suggest you evaluate the potential consequences of doing so. For example, you are following a meal plan that allows you to be flexible, consume most foods in moderation, and not have binging episodes. If you want to continue losing weight and reach 67 kg, you will have to restrict your energy intake.
Patient:	Yes, that's true.
Therapist:	Have you considered the consequences of following a restrictive diet?
Patient:	What do you mean?
Therapist:	For example, how will you handle social situations? I know you go out to eat with your friends twice a week and enjoy spending time with them.
Patient:	I'll eat very little during the day so I can relax in these social situations. Or I'll carefully choose what to eat at the restaurant... Hmm... Maybe it would be better to increase physical activity.
Therapist:	How do you think you would organize your day? Last month, work commitments made it very difficult for you to do 10,000 steps a day.
Patient:	That's true.
Therapist:	Exercising more won't make it easier for you to control what you eat in social situations; if you can only eat 800–1,000 calories a day and you plan to reduce what you eat during the day and do a lot of exercise, at dinner you'll be ravenous. How do you plan to handle the food stimuli you'll be exposed to at the restaurant, the delicious food on the menu and seeing your friends enjoying the food they are eating, for example?
Patient:	I'll have to control myself.
Therapist:	Don't you think excessive control could affect you or have negative consequences?
Patient:	Hmm... Maybe. My friends would probably notice that I wasn't happy and that I wouldn't be much fun. However, it would be worth it in the end.
Therapist:	I also want you to think about whether, in the past, such extreme dietary restriction has worked, and whether there has been any connection between your attempts to rigidly restrict food and the

onset and maintenance of binge episodes (*pointing to the patient's personalized formulation*)

Patient: Yes, that's interesting. In the past, it only worked for a few weeks, and then the binges returned... but now I feel more in control and think I can do it.

The vignette and session transcript above illustrate a common situation in clinical practice where discussing the pros and cons of pursuing the desired weight does not end with the patient's decision to reconsider their goals. In this case, the patient is showing signs of "false hope syndrome", believing that what has never been achievable in the past will be achievable now. It should be noted, however, that the purpose of this intervention is to instil some doubt about the potential risks and drawbacks of overly ambitious weight-loss goals.

Hence, in the last step the therapist should encourage the patient to rewrite the pros and cons of achieving the desired weight as a homework assignment, assessing whether adjusting them to a more realistic and achievable level would be appropriate. This adjustment should consider the issues that may arise if the initial goal is not achieved. Assigned tasks should be reviewed and reassessed during the next session.

Vignette

In the next session, the patient, initially aiming for a desired weight of 67 kg, reported identifying several drawbacks to pursuing that goal. Her list of pros and cons included a negative impact on interpersonal relationships and the risk of binge-eating episodes, experiences she had previously encountered during periods of excessive dietary restriction. She also realized that maintaining extreme and rigid dietary rules to prevent weight regain for the rest of her life would be unrealistic. Considering the benefits already achieved during the weight-loss phase, she decided to focus her efforts on maintaining a weight of around 86 kg.

16.4 Addressing Dysfunctional Primary Goals

The so-called primary goals are those that the patient hopes to achieve through weight loss. These, identified in the third section of the Weight Goals and Primary Goals Questionnaire (see Appendix 5), do not necessarily require significant weight loss or any weight loss at all. Some primary goals, such as improving health and physical fitness, enhancing aesthetic appearance, and altering body shape, can be accomplished through modest weight loss. Others, like improving interpersonal relationships and self-confidence, are not necessarily linked to weight loss [8, 10], and so are considered dysfunctional. The association of psychological and interpersonal goals with weight loss is partly related to the positive stereotyping of thinness in Western society, and the notion of an "ideal" weight [7]. The media promote the alleged association, especially in women, of this physical characteristic with important values such as happiness, control, competence, intelligence and success in relationships.

The first step in addressing dysfunctional primary goals is to review with the patient which goals they have already achieved—likely correlated with weight loss—and those that they have not. The patient should be asked to evaluate whether further weight loss would resolve these "issues", or if different strategies (other than weight loss) might be necessary. Depending on the reasons the patient reports for wanting to lose weight (i.e., their primary goals), there are various interventions the therapist can attempt.

16.4.1 Improving Physical Appearance

Most patients with BED are satisfied with modest weight loss; however, a subgroup maintains a significant level of body dissatisfaction despite the weight loss they have already achieved. In such cases, the therapist should help patients understand that the issue is not their weight (an objective number) but their subjective opinion about their physical appearance. If they can grasp this, they should see that weight loss is not the only solution to their "problem." Alternatively, it may be helpful to suggest that the patient try to develop a different way of thinking about their weight, and consider whether they judge others in the same way that they judge themselves. Conclusions such as "a person's value is not determined by their weight" and "*I can look good at this weight,*" should be elicited, and other solutions for improving physical appearance should be discussed. For example, patients are routinely advised to get a new haircut or buy new clothes and makeup without waiting to reach their desired weight to make these changes. In our clinical experience, this strategy helps most patients reduce dissatisfaction with their bodies and accept a reasonable weight.

16.4.2 Improving Health

One of the most common reasons patients seek treatment for BED associated with clinical obesity, particularly those who are older or have already developed some medical complications such as diabetes, hypertension, cardiovascular diseases, or osteoarthritis, is to improve their health. In most cases, it is unnecessary to address this primary goal directly, as the patient achieves significant health improvement with a 5–10% weight loss and adopting a lifestyle similar to that recommended by the programme. However, if the patient still expresses doubts about progress in health improvement despite reasonable weight loss, it may be helpful to have them repeat the blood tests performed at the beginning of treatment. Generally, the results will show a positive change in key metabolic indicators (blood sugar and lipid profile, liver function, etc.): an objective demonstration of how modest weight loss has significantly improved their health.

16.4.3 Improving Physical Fitness

A common goal for many patients is to improve their physical fitness. In most cases, the goals consist of overcoming some of the difficulties they encounter in their daily lives, such as getting out of breath when climbing the stairs, tying their shoes, or practicing sports. Adopting an active lifestyle, as indicated by CBT for BED, is a strategy that helps improve physical fitness regardless of the total weight lost. Furthermore, an active lifestyle positively affects other primary goals, such as body image, self-confidence, and interpersonal relationships, when exercise is done with others. To demonstrate improved physical fitness objectively, it is useful to ask the patient if, at the weight they have reached, they have reduced some of the physical difficulties they encountered in their daily life at the beginning of the programme.

16.4.4 Improving Interpersonal Relationships

A subgroup of patients seeking weight-loss treatment aims to improve interpersonal relationships, as they irrationally believe that their excess weight is preventing them from making friends or having satisfying relationships. If the patient expresses this motivation for weight loss, the best action is to encourage them to become more socially active immediately, without postponing this goal until they reach their desired weight. The patient should be encouraged to set small, specific, achievable goals (e.g., calling friends and inviting them for a walk or coffee). To address obstacles, the patient should find it helpful to use the proactive problem-solving procedure, which they should already be familiar with (see Chap. 13). It may also be beneficial to ask the patient if they have been avoiding anyone because of their excess weight. If the patient has longstanding interpersonal difficulties (e.g., relational conflicts or interpersonal deficits), they should be directed to a specific psychological treatment to address this issue.

16.4.5 Improving Self-Confidence

In a person with adequate self-esteem, low self-confidence usually stems from simple demoralization associated with weight gain. However, other patients may suffer from long-term low self-esteem. None of these states is necessarily linked to body weight. Still, self-confidence can be improved through various mechanisms addressed by CBT for BED, such as eating control, getting fit, improved physical appearance, and feeling healthier. As with other primary weight-loss goals, it is crucial to suggest that the patient consider trying other strategies, in addition to weight loss, to improve their self-confidence. However, these changes will have a limited effect on individuals who suffer from low self-esteem that is not weight-dependent. In such cases, the patient should be directed to a specific psychological treatment to address the issue.

16.4.6 Making Life Changes

Some patients believe that weight loss will allow them to make significant and beneficial changes in their lives. Examples of changes patients cite include getting a promotion or better job, ending an unsatisfying relationship, beginning a new relationship, or taking up a sport or a new hobby. Typically, these patients tend to postpone the start of these life changes until they reach their desired weight. Again, the strategy should be to suggest to the patient that the desired changes be implemented immediately, without waiting to achieve their primary goal.

16.5 Accepting a Reasonable and Healthy Weight

The final strategy in this type of intervention is to encourage the patient to positively accept their body shape and the weight they have reached through treatment. The emphasis should be on balancing change and acceptance—changing what can be changed (lifestyle) and accepting what cannot be changed (i.e., reaching an "ideal" body shape and weight) [11].

The patient should be helped to accept that extreme weight-control measures, such as rigid dietary restriction and intense physical activity, are counterproductive in the long term. Such extreme and unhealthy behaviours will not help achieve the goal of maintaining an "ideal" shape and weight, and can instead destroy self-confidence and self-esteem. The negative implications of attempting to change what cannot be changed must be balanced with an attempt to consider the current weight and body shape in a more positive light. Ideally, self-acceptance should become an active process of self-affirmation rather than a passive process of resignation or "surrendering to fate" [11]. The goal is to expand the patient's definition and sense of self. To achieve this goal, they should be encouraged to compile a list of personal strengths, independent of their body shape and weight. It may also be helpful to assist the patient in identifying famous individuals who meet current social criteria for physical beauty but have had a miserable life. Sometimes, it is also helpful to ask the patient to give themselves the advice they would give to a friend in a similar situation.

Acceptance of clinical obesity can be facilitated by exploring the origins of the patient's negative beliefs about weight and body shape. Among the factors involved, the therapist should discuss with the patient the societal pressures, prejudices, discrimination, body shaming, and teasing to which people with clinical obesity are often subjected. The patient should be encouraged to think that if people with clinical obesity are discriminated against, it is because they are perceived as belonging to a certain category of people (those who do not fit the ideal), not because of their personality. Therefore, it is not their fault [7].

The ultimate goal of this intervention is not to induce the patient to "love their body" but to reduce excessive emphasis on weight and body shape in their self-evaluation. The patient is not forbidden from being dissatisfied with their body; as already described, such discontent is "normal" in Western culture [12]. A useful analogy for body dissatisfaction is a chronic interpersonal conflict [13] of this kind: "*If you are dissatisfied with your partner, you can decide to leave them, but the only option you have with your body is to make peace with it.*" This involves reaching a compromise and accepting less than what may be considered ideal.

References

1. Calugi S, Marchesini G, El Ghoch M, Gavasso I, Dalle GR. The influence of weight-loss expectations on weight loss and of weight-loss satisfaction on weight maintenance in severe obesity. J Acad Nutr Diet. 2017;117(1):32–8. https://doi.org/10.1016/j.jand.2016.09.001.
2. Dalle Grave R, Melchionda N, Calugi S, Centis E, Tufano A, Fatati G, et al. Continuous care in the treatment of obesity: an observational multicentre study. J Intern Med. 2005;258(3):265–73. https://doi.org/10.1111/j.1365-2796.2005.01524.x.
3. Calugi S, Marchesini G, El Ghoch M, Gavasso I, Dalle Grave R. The association between weight maintenance and session-by-session diet adherence, weight loss and weight-loss satisfaction. Eat Weight Disord. 2020;25(1):127–33. https://doi.org/10.1007/s40519-018-0528-8.
4. Dalle Grave R, Calugi S, Compare A, El Ghoch M, Petroni ML, Tomasi F, et al. Weight loss expectations and attrition in treatment-seeking obese women. Obes Facts. 2015;8(5):311–8. https://doi.org/10.1159/000441366.
5. Dalle Grave R, Calugi S, Molinari E, Petroni ML, Bondi M, Compare A, et al. Weight loss expectations in obese patients and treatment attrition: an observational multicenter study. Obes Res. 2005;13(11):1961–9. https://doi.org/10.1038/oby.2005.241.
6. Dalle Grave R, Sartirana M, Calugi S. Personalized cognitive-behavioural therapy for obesity (CBT-OB): theory, strategies and procedures. Biopsychosoc Med. 2020;14(1):5. https://doi.org/10.1186/s13030-020-00177-9.
7. Dalle Grave R, Sartirana M, El Ghoch M, Calugi S. Treating obesity with personalized cognitive behavioral therapy. Cham: Springer; 2018.
8. Cooper Z, Fairburn CG, Hawker DM. Cognitive-behavioral treatment of obesity: a clinician's guide. Guilford Press; 2003.
9. Dalle Grave R, Sartirana M, El Ghoch M, Calugi S. Module 5: addressing weight-loss dissatisfaction. Treating obesity with personalized cognitive behavioral therapy. Cham: Springer; 2018. p. 117–42.
10. Cooper Z, Fairburn CG. A new cognitive behavioural approach to the treatment of obesity. Behav Res Ther. 2001;39(5):499–511.
11. Wilson GT. Acceptance and change in the treatment of eating disorders and obesity. Behav Ther. 1996;27(3):417–39. https://doi.org/10.1016/S0005-7894(96)80025-6.
12. Rodin J, Silberstein LR, Striegel-Moore RH. Women and weight: a normative discontent. In: Sonderegger TB, editor. Nebraska symposium on motivation: psychology and gender. Lincoln: University of Nebraska Press; 1984. p. 267–307.
13. Cash TF. What do you see when you look in the mirror? New York: Bantam Books; 1995.

Internalized Weight Stigma Module 17

Abstract

Internalized weight stigma arises when a person, applying negative societal weight stereotypes to themselves, develops negative beliefs about themselves and other reactions due to their higher weight. When internalized weight stigma coexists with binge-eating disorder (BED), it must be addressed as it hinders the change because the nature of patients' negative view of themselves and other reactions results in their seeing little or no prospect of being able to control their eating and weight. Furthermore, some patients with internalized weight stigma intermittently strive especially hard to control their eating in pursuit of unrealistic weight goals with a view to reducing their sense of worthlessness. Cognitive behavior therapy (CBT) for BED addresses internalized weight stigma using education and specific cognitive behavioural procedures. When the internalized weight stigma coexists with the overvaluation of shape and weight, the two constructs should be addressed together.

Many patients with BED are self-critical due to their perceived failure to meet their goals of controlling their eating, shape and weight: a form of negative self-evaluation that may be termed "secondary self-criticism". Secondary self-criticism does not generally need to be addressed in treatment because it does not often obstruct change. Furthermore, self-efficacy improves with successful treatment of the eating disorder, even if it has not been explicitly targeted. However, there is a subgroup of patients with "internalized weight stigma" who have a negative core belief about themselves and other reactions due to their weight and shape [1]. This maintains the eating disorder and obstructs change, severely limiting the chances of treatment success unless internalized weight stigma is also overcome. The Internalized Weight Stigma module has been designed for these patients.

R. Dalle Grave et al., *Cognitive Behavior Therapy for Binge Eating Disorder*, https://doi.org/10.1007/978-3-031-71456-6_17

17.1 Description

Internalized weight stigma occurs when a person applies negative societal weight stereotypes to themselves (see Sect. 2.4) and, as a consequence, develops negative beliefs about themselves and other reactions because they perceive that their weight is higher than "normal" [2, 3]. Patients with internalized weight stigma believe that they are lazy, have no willpower, lack self-discipline, and have no self-control. They feel like a failure, think they are ugly and disgusting, and believe that others think the same way. This is a negative view of self-worth not explained by the presence of clinical depression.

17.2 Implications for Treatment

If a patient with BED also has internalized weight stigma, it is particularly difficult for them to enact change in their eating disorder due to two main processes:

1. The nature of a patient's negative view of themselves results in their seeing little or no prospect of their being able to control their eating and weight.
2. The intensity of a patient's internalized stigma leads them to intermittently strive especially hard to control their eating with the aim of achieving unrealistic weight goals and reducing their sense of worthlessness.

17.3 Detecting Internalized Weight Stigma

As reported in Sect. 2.4, internalized weight stigma can theoretically be assessed via the Weight Bias Internalization Scale (WBIS, 10 or 11 items) [2] and/or the Weight Self-Stigma Questionnaire (WSSQ, 12 items) [4]. However, in our clinical experience, neither of these questionnaires enables us to distinguish internalized weight stigma from core low self-esteem, which has the following characteristics [5, 6]:

- It is not condtioned on current performance in the control of eating and weight
- It does not fluctuate (i.e., persistently self-critical)
- The persons see themselves in globally negative terms.

While core low self-esteem entails a stable and pervasive negative self-perception across various life domains, internalized weight bias centres specifically on weight-related self-evaluation, it is reinforced by the omnipresent weight stigma in our society that forms the basis of stereotypes and disparages individuals with higer weight, and it temporarily improves when the individuals is able to lose weight. Internalized weight stigma is characterized by the following two core features:

- Negative view of self and self-worth due to perceived higher weight
- Negative comparisons with others who are "normal" weight

Other features of internalized weight stigma are the presence of pronounced cognitive processing biases (e.g., discounting positive qualities or information, selective attention to information consistent with negative self-view on weight and eating control, over-generalization, dichotomous appraisal of self-worth), safety-seeking strategies, negative emotions, extreme rules related to the control of eating and weight, and the belief that it is impossible to control eating and weight, which undermines the treatment.

It is challenging to identify internalized weight stigma in the presence of clinical depression because the two conditions share many clinical characteristics. We suggest that if there is a coexisting clinical depression that it be addressed first (see Sect. 4.8.1).

17.4 Treatment Strategy

Internalized weight stigma should be a target of treatment if it is concluded that (i) it is contributing to the maintenance of the eating disorder and (ii) it is hindering or impeding treatment. In CBT for BED, internalized weight stigma is addressed using education associated with specific cognitive behavioural procedures. In patients whose internalization of weight stigma coexists with the overvaluation of shape and weight, these procedures should be associated with those described in the Overvaluation of Shape and Weight module.

17.5 Personalized Education

Initially, the therapist should provide personalized education about internalized weight stigma and its contribution to maintaining the patient's eating problem. The key point to stress is that powerful vicious circles operate that serve to entrench both the internalized weight stigma and the binge-eating episodes, as well as dysregulated eating, and overeating. The specific points are described in the following paragraphs.

Environmental stigmatization. People with clinical obesity (see Sect. 4.3.1 and Table 4.4 for the definition) are often the target of denigration and prejudice, and have become part of a socially devalued group [7]. This happens because, in our society, individuals with higher weight tend to be considered lazy, unattractive, lacking willpower and self-discipline, and being responsible for their own condition [8]. Patients should be educated that these stereotypes and/or prejudices are based on ignorance, as several studies have demonstrated that clinical obesity results from a complex interaction between genetic and environmental obesogenic factors [9], and that weight is only partially under the control of the individual. However, it is almost inevitable that patients with higher weight internalize societal weight stigma and apply negative weight stereotypes to themselves, experiencing as they do being identified as belonging to a stigmatized group and being shamed for their weight. Unfortunately, there is very little that we, as therapists, can do to reduce the social stigma of weight that a patient faces. Addressing the individual pressures and social stigma they experience is often challenging. However, the therapist should help the patient become aware of these social pressures and their adverse effects on individuals who do not naturally fall within the BMI range, which is considered "normal." It is also important to help the patient understand that negative societal attitudes toward people with higher weight are unjustified, being merely the result of prejudice and ignorance. Several studies indicate that body weight is determined by a complex interaction between genetic and environmental risk factors. Patients should be edcuated to ask themselves: "Is this my problem or a problem of society at large?". They should be also encouraged to distance themselves from these biases by avoiding adopting the logic of those who hold such views and resisting negative influences. It is also helpful to discuss possible strategies to address social stigma with the patients. These can be as simple as ignoring such attitudes, responding assertively to criticisms about their weight, or more proactive measures, such as writing a letter to a newspaper and/or joining a group that fights prejudice against people with higher weight. If the patients are experiencing weight stigma within their family, the therapist should evaluate, together with the patients, whether it would be helpful to involve significant others in the treatment. In doing so, family members can be educated about weight regulation, the harm caused by weight stigma, and how to eliminate judgmental attitudes toward the patient's eating habits, body shape, and weight.

Negative self-beliefs due to perceived higher weight and other reactions. People with internalized weight stigma think poorly of themselves due to perceived higher weight and how others evaluate them [3]. For example, the belief: "*I am lazy and weak because I cannot control my weight*", is often associated with the belief: "*Others will think I am fat and ugly because I lack self-discipline and willpower*". They have internalized the pervasive societal belief that they themselves are responsible for causing and resolving their higher weight. The belief of not having enough willpower to control eating is self-fulfilling, making eating control difficult, and maintains binge-eating episodes, dysregulated eating, and overeating. Hence, it is often implicated in treatment drop-out. While negative beliefs regarding the reactions of others, more common in those who have experienced weight stigma, may lead the individuals to avoid certain things or places (e.g., travelling or eating in restaurants) because they are scared to do so, this takes away the opportunities for gathering evidence that challenges or debunks their beliefs about others' reactions.

Cognitive biases. These affect the way in which people with internalized weight stigma see the world, their past, and their future. It results in information being filtered so that only negative information based on the perceived higher weight is perceived, thereby confirming their negative view of self. The most common cognitive biases are the following:

- Discounting positive qualities or information about themselves
- Selective attention to information consistent with negative self-view related to the control of weight and eating

- Over-generalization (from any instance of not succeeding at weight and eating control to being a failure)
- All-or-nothing thinking (e.g., "*If I am not normal weight, I must be weak/lazy/greedy.*")

Safety-seeking strategies. Individuals with internalized weight stigma often engage in safety-seeking behaviours to prevent their fears from materializing and to feel more comfortable in anxiety-inducing situations. Everyday scenarios that usually trigger anxiety for these individuals include traveling, being in crowds, going to the beach, eating in a restaurant, having a medical examination, or attending a job interview. One common coping strategy is social avoidance, where individuals distance themselves from others and avoid forming relationships to protect against rejection and stigmatization. Other examples of safety-seeking behaviours include consistently wearing black clothes to camouflage themselves. Additionally, individuals with internalized weight stigma often exhibit hypervigilance and heightened sensitivity to social cues related to weight stigma. Some adopt a submissive role in relationships, viewing themselves as inferior to others, an evolutionary response to perceived social hierarchies. While safety-seeking behaviours can reduce anxiety in the short term and shield individuals from feeling stigmatized, they perpetuate anxiety in the long term. This is because these behaviours prevent the direct testing of fears, allowing untested worries to persist. Moreover, by avoiding certain situations, individuals miss opportunities to gather evidence that could challenge or disconfirm their beliefs about others' negative reactions to their weight. This avoidance maintains negative self-perceptions and reinforces concerns about how others might perceive them.

Problematic rules or expectations. People with internalized weight stigma apply problematic rules to themselves about the control of eating and weight. These rules are intermittently applied to cope with the negative core beliefs that they are unable to control their eating and weight. They are expressed by attempts by having *unrealistic weight and dietary goals* and by adopting *dysfunctional diets*. These rules or expectations are imperative (e.g., "*I* must *become normal weight to be worth anything*"), and place heavy demands on the person. Typical examples are the following:

- "*I have no willpower,*" therefore, "*I have to follow an extreme and rigid diet perfectly.*"
- "*I am fat,*" therefore, "*I have to get down to normal weight.*"
- "*Everyone thinks I have no eating control,*" therefore, "*I always have to eat less than others on social occasions.*"

Experiences of repeated failures, and generalization. Problematic rules regarding eating control and weight goals are inevitably broken, as they are extreme and rigid. Therefore, individuals that have them, having repeated experiences of failure to control eating and being unable to reach their unrealistic weight goals, develop

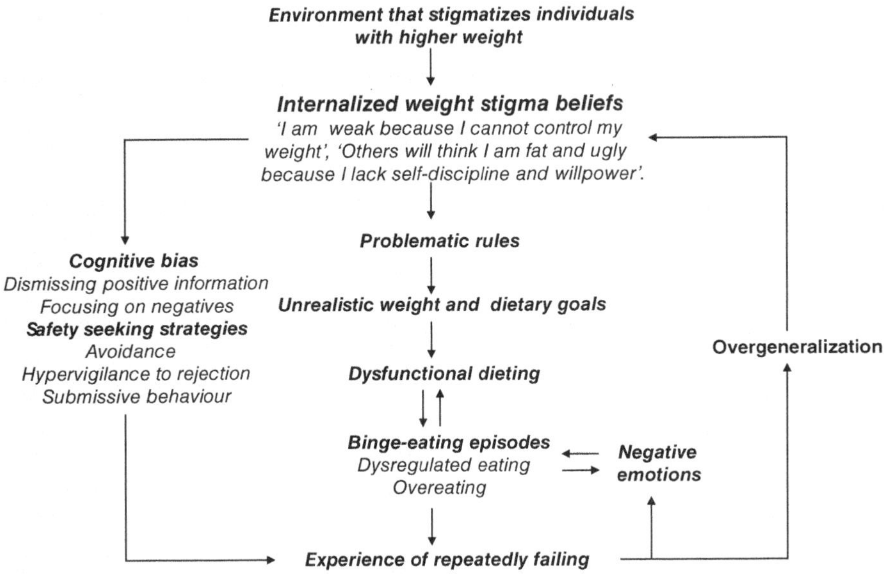

Fig. 17.1 Personal formulation showing how the expressions of internalized weight stigma maintain the eating disorder in a patient with BED

negative emotions (e.g., sadness, shame, guilt, frustration), which trigger new binge eating episodes, dysregulated eating, and overeating, and use cognitive bias to generalize from these perceived failures and see *themselves* as a failure, confirming their negative self-beliefs.

Implications for treatment. Several vicious circles serve to maintain both core internalized weight stigma and BED. Both must be addressed in treatment. Figure 17.1 shows the personal formulation of a patient with BED and internalized weight stigma, which can be used to explain how its expressions maintain the eating-disorder psychopathology.

17.6 Addressing Cognitive Biases

The main cognitive processes that maintain internalized weight stigma and beliefs are addressed using conventional cognitive behavioural procedures [6, 10], as outlined below.

17.6.1 Discounting Positive Qualities

Most patients with internalized weight stigma principally notice their negative qualities while overlooking their positive ones. Identifying positive qualities, however apparently trivial, can help patients understand and achieve a more balanced view of themselves. The procedure uses to address discounting positive qualities has two steps.

Step 1. Asking patients to list their positive attributes, noting their skills and strengths. Patients may find this problematic. It is, therefore, best to start the list in-session. Useful questions to ask to prompt items for the list are as follows:

- What have you achieved in your life so far, however small?
- What skills have you acquired?
- What challenges have you faced?
- What do other people like about or value in you?
- What qualities and attributes do you possess that you value in others?
- What bad qualities do you not have?
- How might a person who cares about you describe you?

Step 2. Encouraging the patient use the above list to raise awareness of their positive attributes daily, independently to their eating control or their weight. For example, the therapist should ask the patient to review the list they drew up in Step 1 and recall specific times when they exhibited qualities that appear on the list. The patient should be invited to:

- Look out for these qualities daily in everyday life and record them.
- Regularly ask themselves, "*What things have gone reasonably well this week?*" and "*Why have they gone well?*", "*How much are the things I have achieved dependent on my eating control or my weight?*" At first, this is best done in-session with the therapist's help, but later on, patients should do this on their own, noting the main points on the back of the day's monitoring record.

17.6.2 Selective Attention

Patients with core internalized weight stigma have selective attention to information that is consistent with their negative beliefs about themselves for their weight and other reactions. The procedure to address selective attention has three steps:

Step 1. Educating patients about selective attention. In general, we all pay particular attention to stimuli that are salient to us. For example, if one buys a new car, one notices many more cars like it. This is not because their number has increased, but because one is paying greater attention to that type of car. The same happens in patients with internalized weight stigma. They look for all their perceived "failures" to control eating and negative comments they received about their weight and eating and find them.

Step 2. Discussing a patient's tendency to look for failure and how this confirms their negative self-belief. The therapist may ask them to give examples (e.g., only remembering times when they overeat and not when they eat regularly, or when they receive criticism at school, not remembering positive feedback).

Step 3. Helping patients become aware of situations in which they engage in selective attention. The goal here is that patients learn to broaden their focus of attention at such times instead of paying particular attention to "failures".

17.6.3 Overgeneralization

Patients with internalized weight stigma tend to view any instance of not succeeding at controlling eating and reaching their unrealistic weight goals as a failure, and then generalize from such failures to being a failure in general. This is addressed via three steps:

Step 1. Fostering patients' awareness of their tendency to overgeneralize from a specific deviation from their eating plan to being "a failure" by helping them to become aware of it occurring.
Step 2. Questioning the basis of the patient's thinking. Ask patients whether they would generalize to their being a wonderful person based on doing one thing well (e.g., sticking to their dietary plan)
Step 3. Encouraging patients to look at the bigger picture and hold back from making global judgements without considering all the evidence.

17.6.4 All-or-Nothing Thinking

People with internalized weight stigma often assess themselves in all-or-nothing terms. They use terms such as "always/never", "everyone/no one", and "everything/nothing" when describing themselves (e.g., "*If I am not always perfectly in control of my diet, that must mean I am weak.*") Such examples of black-and-white appraisals should be addressed via the following three steps:

Step 1. Helping patients to recognize their tendency to appraise themselves in black-and-white terms in the domain of their weight and eating control.
Step 2. Reviewing in detail any justification for such dichotomous assessments of themselves.
Step 3. Encouraging patients to evaluate themselves more flexibly and with greater nuance.

17.7 Addressing Problematic Rules

Problematic rules related to precise control of eating and unrealistic weight goals are common among patients with internalized weight stigma. Beliefs of this kind may be addressed using the strategies and procedures described in the Healthy Weight Loss (Chap. 12), Dysfunctional Dieting (Chap. 14) and Unrealistic Weight Goals (Chap. 16) modules. In addition, patients' thinking can be restructured following four steps:

Step 1. Helping them to recognize and identify their rules on weight and eating control.
Step 2. Helping them consider the impact of their rules on their lives (e.g., relationships, school, leisure activities).
Step 3. Helping them question their current rules on weight and eating control: ask patients (i) where they came from, and (ii) the advantages and disadvantages of following them.

Step 4. Encouraging patients to find alternative rules regarding the control of eating and weight that are more realistic, flexible, and helpful, and to put them into practice. The therapist should remind patients that the new rules will allow them to accept themselves and achieve their life goals.

17.8 Addressing Safety-Seeking Strategies

Safety-seeking strategies should be addressed alongside cognitive interventions. After educating patients on how their actions reinforce internalized weight stigma, they should be guided to understand that facing situations they prefer to avoid is beneficial for testing their predictions and feared negative consequences.

Therapists should assist patients in planning specific behavioural tasks to overcome their fears. This plan, as described in addressing body avoidance in Chap. 15, should involve progressively exposing patients to specific avoided situations, starting with those causing less discomfort (e.g., short traveling, eating in a restaurant, going out with three-quarter-length sleeves instead of long sleeves). Patients should also be encouraged to anticipate the consequences of exposure themselves, record their predictions, and, with the therapist's help, plan how to achieve their goals and face anticipated negative outcomes. During exposure, patients should try to avoid body checking and hypervigilance to social cues related to weight stigma, and instead focus on the positive aspects of the experience.

Finally, therapists should assess the outcome of these attempts and whether the feared negative consequences occurred. They should emphasize the positive aspects, including the patient's achievement in overcoming their reluctance, and re-evaluate with the patient what they have learned from the experience.

17.9 Exploring the Origins of Internalized Weight Stigma

It is helpful to conduct a thorough "historical review", similar to that done when exploring the origins of the eating-disorder mindset (Sect. 18.3), and to reflect with the patient on what may have contributed to their development of internalized weight stigma. This analysis can help the patient understand how their negative beliefs about themselves and other reactions have evolved and persisted. This is best done collaboratively in-session as some patients find the process distressing and may become upset about particular adverse experiences. While it is often difficult to date the onset of internalized weight stigma, the procedure for doing so has the following two steps:

Step 1. Asking patients about events or circumstances that might have contributed to their developing internalized weight stigma. These typically include being exposed to adverse experiences related to eating and weight, such as episodes of body shaming, teasing, or bullying focused on their weight and shape, being excluded or marginalized because of their weight, or not having any friends or other adverse life events.

Step 2. Helping patients re-evaluate past events and experiences. To do this, therapists must help patients examine and question their old appraisals of past experiences and develop new ones.

17.10 Attaining Balanced Self-Worth

The strategies and procedures described above are designed to alter patients' negative views on their worth or value as people. The final step in addressing core internalized weight stigma involves helping patients formulate and accept a more balanced (i.e., less negative) view of themselves. The goal is to get patients to arrive at a more realistic appraisal of their qualities. For example, the judgement: "*I am weak because I'm not losing weight*", may be called into question by a collaborative review of times when they have been strong, especially when it would be acceptable or understandable not to be strong (and bearing in mind that no one is strong all the time). While such a re-appraisal might lead patients to identify areas in which they would still like to make changes, therapists should help patients realize that this does not warrant the (all-or-nothing) conclusion that they are "weak".

This type of re-appraisal should include the notion of "acceptance", and the idea that a balance needs to be struck between "acceptance" and "change". One can change certain aspects of life (e.g., how one eats (within certain limits), the standards one sets for oneself, and how one judges oneself). However, there are other aspects of life that one cannot change (e.g., one's physique and height, one's early experiences), or that can only be changed by a limited extent or with great difficulty (e.g., one's weight in the long-term, one's family, other people). It is necessary to learn to accept those things that cannot be changed, and, as Wilson (2004) has pointed out, doing so is a sign of strength. The goal is for patients to behave in a manner consistent with this new balanced appraisal of themselves, and observe the results of doing so. Examples might include asking for help when previously this was viewed as a sign of weakness; challenging criticism on weight and eating by ignoring it or responding assertively; or being more active, writing a letter to a newspaper and/or joining a group that fights prejudice against people with higher weight with assertive behaviour, for example; or trying to make new friends who do not hold biases about people's weight.

Vignette

The patient, a 25-year-old female with BED and overweight (BMI 26), has made minimal progress, despite having agreed to address the eating disorder alone. In the Review Session at the end of Step One, it emerged that she was harbouring the belief that she was worthless and a failure as a patient because she was "big" and prone to bingeing. In the sessions, she was highly critical of herself, her weight, and her inability to her control eating, expressing the belief that she would never be able to overcome her eating problem. She agreed that she did indeed have negative beliefs about herself, and that this was negatively impacting the treatment. The therapist suggested that they work on overcoming her internalized weight stigma, and she agreed.

Hence, the following sessions covered procedures to address her internalized weight stigma alongside her eating-disorder psychopathology. Specifically, the therapist provided education about societal weight bias, the biological regulation of body weight, and the cognitive biases that seemed to be reinforcing the patient's negative view of herself, and encouraged her to monitor them in real time. This helped the patient to become aware that her most prominent cognitive biases were discounting positive qualities ("*There's nothing good about me.*"), selective attention to minor deviations from her meal plan (which she labelled as "failures"), and overgeneralization ("*I'm weak. I have no willpower.*"). The therapist helped her identify and correct these cognitive biases in real time, and to note and accept the things she did well. This work gradually helped the patient to understand that binge eating was not caused by a lack of willpower, but was being maintained by specific mechanisms, including her negative self-beliefs. She gradually started to question her negative assumptions about herself and become more active in addressing the mechanisms maintaining her binge-eating episodes because she began to believe that it was possible to overcome her eating problem.

At the end of the treatment, her BED was in remission, and she recognized that her previously held view of being worthless and a failure because she had a higher weight was erroneous. She decided to face life accepting her body shape and herself.

References

1. Durso LE, Latner JD, White MA, Masheb RM, Blomquist KK, Morgan PT, et al. Internalized weight bias in obese patients with binge eating disorder: associations with eating disturbances and psychological functioning. Int J Eat Disord. 2012;45(3):423–7. https://doi.org/10.1002/eat.20933.
2. Durso LE, Latner JD. Understanding self-directed stigma: development of the weight bias internalization scale. Obesity. 2008;16(Suppl 2):S80–6. https://doi.org/10.1038/oby.2008.448.
3. Ratcliffe D, Ellison N. Obesity and internalized weight stigma: a formulation model for an emerging psychological problem. Behav Cogn Psychother. 2015;43(2):239–52. https://doi.org/10.1017/S1352465813000763.
4. Lillis J, Luoma JB, Levin ME, Hayes SC. Measuring weight self-stigma: the weight self-stigma questionnaire. Obesity. 2010;18(5):971–6. https://doi.org/10.1038/oby.2009.353.
5. Fairburn CG, Cooper Z, Shafran R, Bohn K, Hawker D. Clinical perfectionism, core low self-esteem and interpersonal problems. In: Fairburn CG, editor. Cognitive behavior therapy and eating disorders. New York: Guilford Press; 2008. p. 47–123.

6. Fennell M. Overcoming low self-wsteem. London: Constable & Robinson; 2009.
7. Puhl R, Brownell KD. Bias, discrimination, and obesity. Obes Res. 2001;9(12):788–805. https://doi.org/10.1038/oby.2001.108.
8. Brownell KD, Puhl RM, Schwartz MB, Rudd L. Weight bias: nature, consequences, and remedies. New York: Guilford Press; 2005.
9. Masood B, Moorthy M. Causes of obesity: a review. Clin Med (Lond). 2023;23(4):284–91. https://doi.org/10.7861/clinmed.2023-0168.
10. Fennell MJ. Overcoming low self-esteem: a self-help guide using cognitive behavioural techniques. 2nd ed. London: Constable & Robinson; 2016.

Setbacks and Mindsets Module

18

Abstract

Towards the end of Step Two, if the treatment is going well, the patient should experience a progressive reduction in the intensity of their concerns about eating control associated with the remission of binge-eating episodes and dysregulated eating and overeating. This is the point at which the Setbacks and Mindsets module should be introduced. Patients should be informed that setbacks (i.e., an episode of binge eating, dysregulated eating, overeating, body checking, or dysfunctional dieting) are inevitable. However, these setbacks are often preceded by reactivation of the "mindset" typical of the eating disorder, that is, the way of thinking about the eating disorder and, in particular, the overvaluation of shape and weight or the lack of attention to eating behaviour and weight. Patients are also informed that if addressed immediately, relapse will be avoided. Having educated the patients on mindsets, the procedures of this module are designed to help the patient identify stimuli that are likely to reactivate the eating-disorder mindset, spot setbacks early on, and displace the mindset.

Towards the end of Step Two, if things have been done well, the patient should be experiencing a progressive reduction in the intensity of their concerns about eating control associated with the remission of binge-eating episodes and dysregulated eating and overeating. At this point in the treatment, patients should also be informed that setbacks are inevitable, but that the strategies and procedures in the Setbacks and Mindsets module are designed to help them take immediate action, and therefore prevent the occasional lapse from becoming a relapse.

R. Dalle Grave et al., *Cognitive Behavior Therapy for Binge Eating Disorder*,
https://doi.org/10.1007/978-3-031-71456-6_18

18.1 Education on Setbacks and Mindsets

Setbacks occur whenever one or more expressions of the eating disorder psychopathology reappear (e.g., an episode of binge eating, dysregulated eating, overeating, body checking, or dysfunctional dieting). Although it might seem that they return "out of the blue", they are in fact preceded by reactivation of the "mindset" typical of the eating disorder, that is, the way of thinking about the eating disorder and, in particular, the overvaluation of shape and weight or the lack of attention to eating behaviour and weight.

The first step in learning to deal effectively with such lapses is to understand what we mean by "mindset" [1]. Hence the patient should be educated on the matter, perhaps using the following analogy: "*If you compare your mind to a music app, you might have several playlists for different occasions: one that you listen to when you are studying, one when you are having fun with friends, one when you are driving or working out, etc. Each playlist corresponds to a characteristic mental state, or 'mindset' that is activated under specific circumstances.*"

The therapist should explain to the patient that as they have an "eating disorder" playlist, or mindset. This mindset typically [2, 3]:

- Filters external and internal stimuli in a specific way (e.g., predominantly noticing thin people) such that it creates its own, non-objective, reality.
- Leads to the adoption characteristic behaviours (e.g., binge-eating episodes, adoption of rigid and extreme dietary rules).

It is also very difficult to dislodge, causing the patient to be "locked in" to this frame of mind. In this situation, other mindsets cannot activate in circumstances that require them (e.g., at work, instead of activating the "work" playlist, the "eating disorder" playlist stays on) by producing continuous concerns about eating that drown out other thoughts.

Continuing this analogy, the therapist elucidates that in the advanced phases of treatment, once the core maintenance mechanisms of the eating disorder have been dismantled, patients are likely to observe instances when the eating-disorder mindset is temporarily silenced, and they can once again hear the right playlist for the circumstances. At this point, the patient is likely to find themselves oscillating between states of being "in" or "out" of their eating-disorder mindset. However, particularly in the early stages, these "out" periods tend to be fleeting, since it is relatively easy for the eating-disorder mindset to be reactivated. Once reactivated, eating-disorder features swiftly resurface, including binge eating, dysfunctional dieting, body checking, and body avoidance (refer to Fig. 18.1).

Even though the propensity for the eating-disorder mindset to reactivate diminishes over time with the treatment, there is still a considerable chance of this occurrence, especially in the initial stages of recovery. Consequently, the therapist should encourage patients to recognize this phase as an opportune moment to develop skills for effectively managing and controlling the eating-disorder mindset.

Vignette

The patient is a 35-year-old woman who, after a period free from binge-eating episodes, came to a session very frustrated because she had experienced a binge the day before. From a collaborative review of her monitoring record, it emerged that she had begun to worry about her weight after going to a store and not finding her size in a dress she liked. The next day, she resumed body checking (i.e., scrutinizing the shape of her legs and buttocks), which she had previously suspended in the Overvaluation of Shape and Weight module. This was accompanied by her concerns about her body intensifying, and her deciding to eliminate carbohydrates to lose weight. On the day before the session, after eating a slice of cake offered by a colleague in the office to celebrate her birthday, she became worried about having ruined her diet, and after lunch, she had a binge-eating episode in the afternoon. After reviewing the relevant monitoring records with the patient to help her reconstruct this sequence of events, the therapist took the opportunity to educate her on setbacks, the eating-disorder mindset, and how to control it in the future.

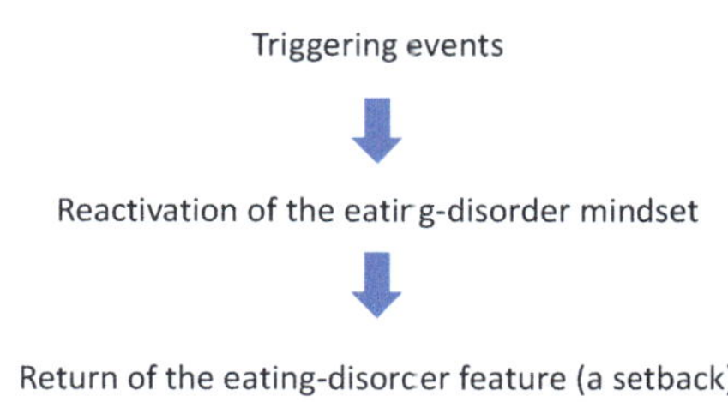

Fig. 18.1 Sequence of events leading to a setback

18.2 Strategy for Controlling the Eating-Disorder Mindset

Having educated the patients on mindsets, the therapist should explain the main CBT strategy for controlling the eating-disorder mindset, which includes learning how to [2, 4]:

- Identify stimuli that are likely to reactivate the eating-disorder mindset
- Spot setbacks early on
- Displace the mindset
- N.B. We advise not introducing this strategy in the early phases of the treatment because, at that point, the patients' eating-disorder mindset is firmly locked in place, and they have no other state to compare it with.

18.2.1 Identifying Stimuli Likely to Reactivate the Eating-Disorder Mindset

The common triggers for eating-disorder mindset reactivation are the following:

- Events related to weight and body shape (e.g., weight fluctuations, tight clothing, checking in the mirror, receiving critical comments from others)
- Events related to eating (e.g., breaking a dietary rule, eating "too much", feeling full)
- Adverse events in general (e.g., negative events in general, interpersonal conflicts)
- Low mood (e.g., secondary to adverse circumstances or clinical depression)

The therapist should recommend that the patient monitor the types of stimuli that are most likely to trigger their eating disorder in real time. In many cases, such in-the-moment awareness is sufficient for them to overcome the influence of these stimuli.

18.2.2 Spotting Setbacks Early On

The therapist should communicate to patients that there will inevitably be instances in which the eating-disorder mindset resurfaces. In such cases, it is crucial to promptly recognize the initial shifts in eating behaviours—such as dysfunctional dietary restrictions and excessive body checking, which we call the "relapse signature". Understanding that these changes serve as early warning signs for the resurgence of their eating-disorder mindset is paramount. Indeed, if the eating-disorder mindset is not promptly addressed (within a day or two), the primary maintenance mechanisms will begin solidifying its reinstatement, making it exceedingly challenging to displace. Conversely, recognizing and addressing the eating-disorder mindset as soon as it reactivates makes the displacement process much more manageable.

18.2.3 Displacing the Eating-Disorder Mindset

In preparation for the inevitable reactivation of the eating-disorder mindset, patients should be taught to (i) "do the right thing" (usually the opposite of the behaviour driven by the eating-disorder mindset) and (ii) engage in distracting, preferably interpersonal, activities.

"Doing the right thing" entails embracing behaviours that align with the principles learned in treatment to counteract the influence of the eating-disorder mindset. Essentially, patients should do the opposite of what the eating-disorder mindset dictates. Engaging in enjoyable or engrossing activities can serve as a powerful means of overriding urges. While activities involving other people (such as going out with a friend) are generally most effective for this purpose, regrettably, they tend to pose significant challenges for individuals with eating disorders. Nevertheless, patients must recognize that overcoming these challenges is a crucial step toward permanently displacing the eating-disorder mindset. Setbacks can be viewed as valuable opportunities to do so. They offer real chances to practice identifying eating-disorder mindset reactivation and employing the appropriate strategies to address it. These efforts can then be reviewed collaboratively with the therapist, allowing any obstacles to be addressed with their support, until patients develop the confidence to navigate future setbacks effectively on their own.

Through consistent practice, patients develop a growing proficiency in displacing their mindset. The significance of practice cannot be overstated, and successfully displacing the eating-disorder mindset instils a sense of mastery over setbacks. While vulnerability to setbacks typically diminishes over time as a general trend, it remains crucial for patients to preserve this skill, as it may prove valuable in the face of potential challenges in the future.

18.3 Exploring the Origins of the Eating-Disorder Mindset

Towards the end of Step Two, it can be beneficial to reflect with the patient on what may have contributed to the onset of binge-eating episodes. This analysis can help the patient understand how their eating disorder evolved, and why its initial positive functions may no longer be relevant as they recover. It is important to note that the causes of eating disorders are not entirely understood, so the conclusions drawn from this analysis should be considered speculative rather than definitive. With a view to attaining a better understanding of their psychopathology, the patient should be asked to consider three periods of their life:

1. Before the eating disorder (i.e., up to a point 12 months before its onset)
2. The 12 months preceding the onset of the eating disorder
3. From the onset of the eating disorder to the present day

For each period, patients should reflect on whether any events or circumstances might have influenced the onset of binge-eating episodes. By organizing their ideas on a "life chart" (see Fig. 18.2), hypotheses about the development and evolution of their eating disorder can be collaboratively formulated.

Typically, events up to 12 months before the onset involve adverse and traumatic experiences, personal or parental depression, other mental health disorders, personal or parental higher weight, and low self-esteem. Events occurring in the 12 months before the onset tend to involve general life stressors (e.g., academic or work failures, the end of a romantic relationship, starting a new school or job, moving house, parental separation, grief, or receiving negative comments about weight or body shape, adoption of dysfunctional diets). The third period is invariably characterized by the gradual emergence of the various maintenance mechanisms highlighted in the personal formulation, rendering the eating disorder self-sustaining.

Time period	*Events and situations*
Up to 12 months before the onset of the eating disorder	*Childhood overweight* *Teasing about weight and body shape from classmates* *Mother with depression* *Social anxiety*
The 12 months before the onset of the eating disorder	*Adoption of a strict diet and loss of 10 kg in two months*
From the onset of the eating disorder until today	*Emergence of binge-eating and disordered eating, with regain of all lost weight (at age 17)* *Relationship ending(at age 18)* *Starting university (at age 19)* *Increased frequency of binge-eating* *Attempts at dysfunctional diets (ketogenic diet, fasting, meal replacements, etc.)* *Further weight gain* *Depression (start of psychotherapy and antidepressants at age 20)* *Dropped out of university*

Fig. 18.2 Example of a life chart of a patient with BED

If conducted in the later stages of the programme, when the patient experiences more extended periods without binge-eating episodes, this analysis, in addition to "normalizing" the experience—acknowledging that it was inevitable given the circumstances—can aid the patient in further distancing them from the eating-disorder mindset.

References

1. Teasdale JD. Metacognition, mindfulness and the modification of mood disorders. Clin Psychol Psychother. 1999;6(2):146–55. https://doi.org/10.1002/(sici)1099-0879(199905)6:2<146::Aid-cpp195>3.0.Co;2-e.
2. Fairburn CG. Cognitive behavior therapy and eating disorders. New York: Guilford Press; 2008.
3. Dalle Grave R, Calugi S. Cognitive behavior therapy for adolescents with eating disorders. New York: Guilford Press; 2020.
4. Dalle Grave R, Calugi S. A young person's guide to cognitive behaviour therapy for eating disorders. London: Routledge; 2024.

Maintenance Preparation Module

19

Abstract

The final part of Step Two in cognitive behaviour therapy (CBT) for binge-eating disorder (BED) consists of three appointments, each separated by a 2-week interval. While the session structure remains constant, the focus gradually shifts towards future-oriented goals, of which there are three. The first is assessing progress made and the residual features to address. This involves reviewing any perceived positive changes in physical and psychosocial well-being associated with binge management (and weight in those who have undertaken weight loss), and jointly assessing which eating disorder features remain to be tackled during the maintenance. The second goal of maintenance preparation is to identify programme procedures to phase out (e.g., using the monitoring records and in-session collaborative weighing), and those that should be continued (e.g., regular eating, weekly weighing at home, proactive problem-solving, binge-eating analyses, daily step counts). The third goal is to introduce specific procedures to prevent relapse and ensure weight maintenance. This is achieved by collaboratively constructing a long-term maintenance plan, which should contain personalized advice on which residual feature of BED and weight maintenance (if indicated) to address and, at the same time, how to minimize the risk of relapse (e.g., reminders on how to deal with triggers and setbacks).

The last part of Step Two of CBT for BED consists of three appointments spaced 2 weeks apart. The structure of the session remains unchanged, but the sessions progressively focus more on the future and have the following objectives:

- Assessing progress made and the residual eating-disorder features to address
- Identifying which procedures to discontinue and which to continue
- Introducing relapse-prevention strategies
- Constructing a maintenance plan

R. Dalle Grave et al., *Cognitive Behavior Therapy for Binge Eating Disorder*, https://doi.org/10.1007/978-3-031-71456-6_19

Patients who have addressed weight loss are also educated on the procedures to adopt to maintain body weight.

19.1 Assessing Progress Made and Residual Features to Address

Reviewing changes in physical and psychosocial well-being associated with binge management (and weight in those who have undertaken weight loss) is an effective way to introduce the topic of long-term maintenance. It helps the patient appreciate the importance of preventing relapse. The therapist should ask the patient to compare their current lifestyle, physical condition, and health with how they were before starting the treatment. In most cases, patients report having adopted a healthy diet and an active lifestyle, in addition to cessation of binge eating, dysregulated eating, and overeating; improved sleep; reduced fatigue and joint pain; and improved physical fitness. For patients with clinical obesity who have achieved reasonable weight loss, physical improvements can be confirmed by normalized blood test results and a reduction in medication used to treat related comorbidities (e.g., hypertension, diabetes, dyslipidaemia), and/or improvement in physical fitness. The therapist should also remember to enquire whether remission of binge eating has been associated with any *psychosocial* improvements. Many patients report enhanced self-esteem, mood, and body image, reduced avoidance of situations due to weight, and increased confidence during social occasions.

In addition to the clinical interview, the same questionnaires administered at the beginning of the treatment (e.g., EDE-Q, BSI, CIA, SF-36, and WBIS) should be filled in again. The goal is to show the patient their improvements in black and white, and to underline that they have played the main role in achieving those results.

Subsequently, the therapist and patient should jointly assess which eating-disorder features remain to be tackled during the maintenance phase. A review of the patient's formulation will highlight which residual maintenance mechanisms should be addressed.

19.2 Identifying Procedures to Discontinue and Continue

At this stage, it is advisable to stop using the monitoring records. It is neither realistic nor appropriate to ask the patient to continue monitoring indefinitely. It is more advantageous for the interruption to occur when the patient is still undergoing active treatment, so that the therapist is available to help them analyze the consequences. Many patients are relieved at the idea of suspending monitoring, while others, albeit a minority, report concerns about the possibility of no longer feeling in control, and not being able to observe and analyze what they are doing. The therapist should stress that, at this point in the process, they have acquired the skills necessary to be more aware of their behaviours, thoughts, and emotions and, therefore, the monitoring records, despite being indispensable in the early stages of the programme, are now surplus to requirements ("*If you know a song by heart, you don't need to study the notes any more.*"). The therapist should, however, encourage the patient to remain vigilant, and stay alert for any changes in their eating habits and any other aspect of the eating disorder that they have addressed during treatment (e.g., dietary rules, events, and emotions that influence eating, body checking, body avoidance).

Another procedure to interrupt during the session is collaborative weighting. The patients will have to weigh themselves at home in the same way they have been doing collaboratively (i.e., on a set day, once a week, with the number entered on a weight graph and weight interpreted in the context of the last 4 weeks). However, in the first few weeks, weighing should be done both in-session and at home twice, to calibrate the two sets of scales. After that, patients should begin to weigh themselves only at home. In-session weighing should cease at this time. The therapist should review the patients' weight graph with them while the sessions are ongoing and deal with any difficulties. The patient should also be asked to continue completing the EPCLI-BED immediately after the weekly weighing. This will allow them to identify any difficulties that arise each week, and prompt rapid intervention.

The patient should also be asked which strategies and procedures have been particularly helpful in enabling them to overcome some aspects of their eating disorder. These should be continued, even after the end of treatment, to minimize the risk of relapse. In our experience, the procedures that most patients find it useful to continue are the following:

- Regular eating
- Weekly weighing
- Proactive problem-solving
- Binge-eating analyses
- Daily step counting

19.3 Introducing Relapse Prevention Strategies

A primary focus in this phase of the treatment is placed on mitigating the risk of relapse in the future. This extends the insights gained about overcoming setbacks in the Setbacks and Mindsets module (see Chap. 18). Patients are explicitly reminded that binge-eating lapses are not uncommon after treatment. It is crucial to emphasize the significance of promptly and effectively addressing setbacks to prevent potential relapse. In this regard, the therapist needs to ensure that the patient grasps three key points:

1. *Realistic expectations*. Patients should perceive their eating disorder as an Achilles' heel, acknowledging that the eating-disorder mindset may resurface in certain situations. However, as learned in the Setbacks and Mindsets module, patients can "head it off at the pass", and should apply the strategies and procedures they have learned to avoid falling into a negative mindset

2. *High-risk situations*. Various situations increase the risk of relapse, such as engaging in dysfunctional dieting, experiencing changes in shape and weight, encountering stressful circumstances, or developing clinical depression. The important thing is for a patient to recognize the danger early on and take evasive action.
3. *Lapses vs. relapses*. It's fundamental to distinguish lapses (setbacks) from relapses. Patients should understand that their reactions to setbacks determine the course of action. Viewing setbacks as "lapses" instead of full-scale "relapses" helps avert a self-fulfilling prophecy. Hence, patients should be encouraged to adopt a proactive "can-do" attitude that fosters effective problem-solving, rather than a hopeless passive stance.

With these factors in mind, a personalized plan for addressing setbacks should be collaboratively formulated. This should comprise two components:

1. *Spotting setbacks promptly*, steering clear of wishful thinking, decentring from the eating-disorder mindset as soon as possible by "doing the right thing" and engaging in activities, preferably interpersonal, that will shift the mindset.
2. *Addressing the trigger.* Patients are encouraged to take a thoughtful "time out" to contemplate the potential roots of the setback. Subsequently, they should employ the problem-solving procedures acquired during treatment to effectively address and mitigate the trigger's impact on their progress.

19.4 Introducing Weight Maintenance Procedures

These procedures are principally reserved for the patients who, in Step Two, have lost weight through the strategies and procedures described in the Healthy Weight Loss module. However, with some adaptation they can also be helpful to other patients recovering from BED.

19.4.1 Education about Weight Maintenance

The patient should be provided education on weight maintenance covering three main topics [1]: (i) maintaining weight is more challenging than losing weight; (ii) some individuals can sustain long-term weight loss; and (ii) specific skills need to be learned and practiced to maintain weight.

Maintaining weight is more difficult than losing weight for several reasons:

- Acceptance of a weight that was previously deemed unacceptable is necessary.
- Unlike weight loss, which has a defined duration, weight maintenance is an indefinite, lifelong process.
- Individuals often receive little encouragement from significant others during weight maintenance, and may even face criticism for not attempting further weight loss.

- Positive outcomes of weight loss can be assessed weekly, while evaluating weight maintenance requires months or years.
- During weight loss, the goal is improvement (e.g., weight, health, appearance), whereas during weight maintenance, the objective is preserving the results achieved.
- If a large amount of weight has been lost, there is increased biological pressure to regain weight

The therapist should emphasize that weight regain after weight loss is an insidious process, significantly different from what generally happens in substance misuse [1]. For instance, someone who has quit smoking knows that a single cigarette might lead to relapse and is therefore careful to avoid any transgression to maintain lasting abstinence. However, in weight maintenance, except for cases with frequent binge-eating episodes, the initial steps toward relapse are usually less apparent. In many cases, the relapse process starts with small but persistent changes in eating habits (e.g., consuming high-fat foods, snacking) or physical activity routines (e.g., fewer than 10,000 steps per day). These changes may not necessarily result in an immediate weight gain, as gaining 1 kg requires consuming approximately 7,000 kcal more than those burned. This fact may lead individuals to develop false confidence in eating more and moving less without gaining weight. Even when there is a regain of 2 kg, patients are often unaware that relapse is occurring, thinking they can easily lose this weight whenever they want (the so-called "false hope syndrome"). However, this amount of regained weight often signals that old habits have been reactivated and reinstated for a persistent period, and the patient is already on a path that almost inevitably leads to their gradually regaining all the lost weight. This is why CBT for BED places so much importance during the weight maintenance phase on patients learning to pay attention to early signs of relapse (i.e., changes in eating and/or physical activity routines), referred to as setbacks. They need to become experts at nipping deleterious habits in the bud, even before their weight begins to rise. In short, patients must be taught when and how to get back on track.

The therapist should also reinforce the notion that it *is* possible for individuals to maintain their weight loss in the long term by describing the results of the National Weight Control Registry (NWCR) analysis to the patient. That study was designed to follow individuals (18 years or older) who lost at least 13.6 kg (30 pounds) of weight and maintained it for at least 1 year. Over 10,000 people participated in the study, annually completing questionnaires about their current weight, eating, and exercise habits, and behavioural strategies for weight maintenance. In 2014, the study reported observations based on self-reported weight loss and behavioural change data at 10 years in 2,886 participants, primarily recruited through newspapers and magazines. The average weight loss reported for these participants was 31.3 kg at baseline, 23.8 kg at 5 years, and 23.1 kg at 10 years Notably, 87% of participants maintained a weight loss of at least 10% after 5 and 10 years. The therapist should emphasize that the exceptional NWCR data show that long-term maintenance of lost weight is achievable. The therapist should inform the patient that those who maintained weight in the NWCR study adopted the following behavioural strategies [2]:

1. Engaging in high levels of physical activity (about 1 hour per day)
2. Following a low-energy, low-fat diet
3. Having breakfast every day
4. Weighing themselves regularly
5. Maintaining appropriate eating habits on weekdays and at weekends

Furthermore, the likelihood of long-term success increased in those who maintained weight for 2 years or more.

The therapist should inform patients that, unfortunately, the NWCR study was not designed to answer the central question: why some individuals can continue practicing weight-control behaviours and maintain weight loss in the long term while others cannot. Some have suggested that the biological pressure for individuals to eat more to restore their original weight is the driving force behind weight regain (the set-point theory) [3]. In contrast, others have argued it is exposure to an environment that promotes overeating and sedentary behaviours [4]. In any event, the NWCR study clearly shows that many people *can* overcome these pressures in the long term and maintain significant weight loss through lifestyle modification.

If not entirely due to biological pressures, the therapist should suggest that cognitive mechanisms interacting with specific diet and physical activity changes will likely play a fundamental role in long-term weight maintenance. The complex behaviours involved in lifestyle modification—in this case, the adoption and practice of strategies necessary for weight loss and maintenance—are partly influenced by conscious cognitive processes. Our research, for example, has indicated that weight maintenance is associated with greater satisfaction with achieved weight loss and its related benefits [5]. In contrast, a decrease in satisfaction with weight loss during the weight-loss phase is correlated with long-term weight regain [6]. These findings suggest that cognitive processes strongly influence the likelihood of persisting with weight maintenance behaviours. Specifically, for long-term success, it is necessary to appreciate the achieved weight loss—even if lower than expected or desired—and to develop a long-term weight-control mindset.

The patient should be informed that, after about 6 months (in most cases), weight loss tends to slow down and eventually stop. For this reason, CBT for BED initiates the weight-maintenance phase at 24 weeks, focusing on reducing the risk of relapse. It is important to emphasize that time and effort will be required to learn how to maintain lost weight and avoid relapse. During the maintenance phase, it is essential to halt any attempts at further weight loss, as this is incompatible with acquiring the cognitive and behavioural skills necessary for long-term weight maintenance.

19.4.2 Actively Involving the Patient in the Decision to Start Weigh Maintenance

After examining the benefits derived from weight loss and instructing the patient on weight maintenance, the next step is to collaboratively assess the pros and cons of initiating it. The therapist should ask the patient to reflect on their reasons for and against starting weight maintenance. As always, it is advisable to begin by asking the patient to list the cons, and whether continuing to pursue weight loss would provide benefits they fear missing out on or do not want to give up. Subsequently, the patient should be encouraged to evaluate the pros. At this stage, the therapist should prompt them to consider that the failure of previous weight-loss attempts may have been due, in part, to not learning and practicing weight-maintenance skills. The list of pros and cons and the conclusions the patient draws from this discussion should be transcribed into a table (see the example in Table 19.1).

If, despite this analysis, the patient is reluctant to start the maintenance phase, the therapist should temporarily accept their decision but emphasize the risks of continuing to pursue weight loss. In these cases, the therapist should dedicate subsequent sessions to intensifying efforts to help them address obstacles to accepting weight maintenance using the procedure described in Chap. 16.

19.4.3 Addressing Questions and Concerns about Starting Weight Maintenance

It is always important to ask the patient if they have any doubts or questions about starting the weight maintenance phase. Here are some examples:

Patient: I'm a bit worried about starting weight maintenance. In the past, I always regained the weight I had lost.

Therapist: It's not uncommon for you to be concerned about weight maintenance because, as you know from your experience and as we discussed earlier, it's the most challenging part of the treatment.

Table 19.1 Example pros and cons of starting weight maintenance table

Reasons not to start weight maintenance	Reasons to start weight maintenance
I want to lose another 10 kg	I haven't lost weight for 4 weeks
I am still fat	I have already gained several benefits from weight loss
I will be more attractive and happier if I lose more weight	In the past, I have never tried to maintain weight and have always regained lost weight
If I better control my diet, I will lose more weight, and then I will be more satisfied	I don't know how to maintain weight—I'm always either losing weight or putting it on
Conclusions: I want to start weight maintenance because I have already gained numerous benefits from weight loss, I no longer binge, and I need to learn how to maintain weight	

However, this programme has been specifically designed to help you develop the skills you need to maintain weight long term and prevent relapse in your eating disorder. Moreover, you can use your past experiences to help you identify early signs of relapse and prevent weight regain.

Patient: I know starting weight maintenance is important, but my husband told me I still need to lose more weight.

Therapist: I'm glad you agree on the importance of starting weight maintenance. Perhaps we could meet with your husband to explain why you should begin it and ask for his support.

Patient: Yes, I think that's a good idea.

Patient: What should I do if I start having binge episodes and gaining weight?

Therapist: Good question. During treatment, you've already developed skills to manage residual binge episodes. In the maintenance phase, you'll learn specific skills to prevent weight regain and get back to an acceptable weight-maintenance range if that were to happen.

Patient: Could I change my mind and decide to lose more weight later, for example, in about a month?

Therapist: Certainly. You're free to decide what to do. However, I don't think that would be a good idea because you need time to learn and implement the skills necessary for weight maintenance.

Patient: I feel like I can lose more weight. Why should I start maintaining it?

Therapist: If you're confident you can lose more weight, you could continue the weight-loss phase for a couple of months. However, before making that decision, we should carefully evaluate the pros and cons of delaying the start of the weight-maintenance phase. Whatever your decision, be aware that weight maintenance is an integral part of the treatment, and it will need to be undertaken sooner or later if you want to maintain the weight successfully.

Vignette

The patient, a 39-year-old single, female nurse, achieved a weight loss of 13 kg after 24 weeks of treatment (from 87 to 74 kg). Furthermore, she had stopped binge eating after just 4 weeks. She reported that the weight loss she had achieved so far made her feel physically and psychologically much better. Additionally, she had been receiving many compliments from friends and started a romantic relationship. Despite these benefits, she was reluctant to start weight maintenance because her goal was to reach a "normal" weight. However, over the last month, her weight had remained stable. After receiving information about the need to learn and practice weight-maintenance skills and reassessing the failure of previous weight-loss attempts, in which she had never experienced a period of weight maintenance and had always regained weight and resumed binge-eating episodes, she agreed to start the maintenance phase. After 48 weeks of maintenance, she weighed 72 kg, which she maintained by adopting a healthy and flexible pattern of eating, and reported no binge-eating episodes. In the interview conducted at the end of the treatment, she noted that it had been a good decision to stop attempting further weight loss and to focus solely on maintenance. She expressed great appreciation for her current lifestyle, physical fitness (being able to jog for 45 minutes without feeling tired), and acceptance of her body shape.

19.4.4 Establishing Weekly Weighing at Home and the Weight-Maintenance Range

Research has shown that one of the most important procedures for long-term weight maintenance is regular weighing, and individuals who cease to do so tend to regain all the weight they have lost [2]. It has been suggested that regular weighing has the potential to allow individuals to promptly detect an energy imbalance before these changes lead to substantial weight regain [7]. Regular weighing, commonly once a week, has also been reported by most of those in the National Weight Control Registry (NWCR) who have successfully maintained their lost weight [8]. Therefore, the therapist should inform patients that weighing themselves once a week, initiated in Step One of the treatment, is a key procedure for weight maintenance and should become a lifelong habit, akin to bathing or tooth brushing.

To this end, the therapist should provide the patient with a new blank copy of the weight graph (see Fig. A2.1 in Appendix 2) plotting two red lines to represent a weight maintenance range of 2 kg above and below the patient's current weight (i.e., the average of the last 4 weeks) (Fig. 19.1). A 4 kg range was chosen because weight tends to fluctuate due to normal variations in body hydration status [9].

In addition to interpreting weight fluctuation over 4 weeks rather than a single reading (as in Step One), the patient should be instructed to pay attention to the following two situations in interpreting the weight maintenance chart (see Fig. 19.1):

1. *Weight moving outside the maintenance range*. If the weight increases above the maximum acceptable range, the patient should immediately implement a pre-prepared action plan to get back on track. Similarly, if their weight drops below the maintenance range minimum, the patient needs to assess whether this weight loss was intentional. If intentional, further weight loss should be discouraged because the goal is to learn to maintain weight, not lose it: a necessary aspect for long-term success. However, if the weight loss was unintentional, calorie intake should be adjusted to keep the weight within the maintenance range.
2. *Weight continuously rising*. In this case, the patient is advised to evaluate whether the weight gain is related to normal weight fluctuations or is the beginning of a weight regain trend. To get to the bottom of this issue, the patient should con-

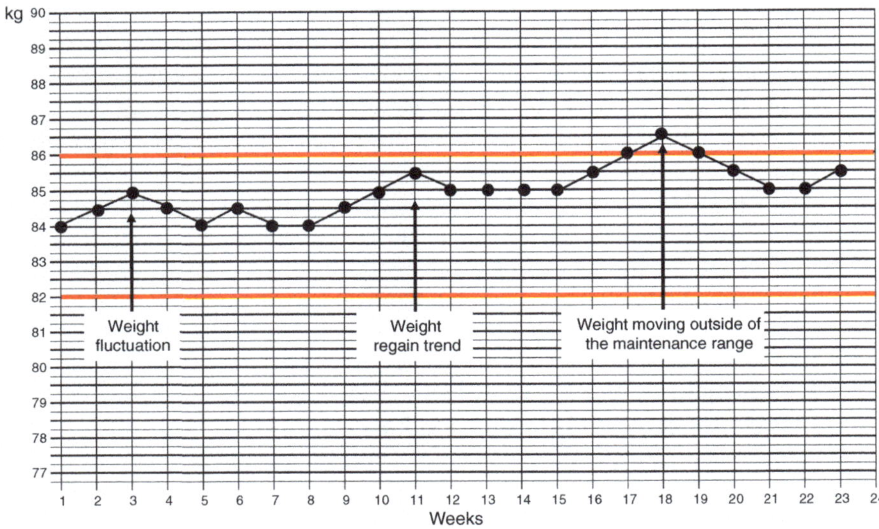

Fig. 19.1 An example of a weight-maintenance graph showing weight fluctuation, weight gain trend, and weight going outside the effective maintenance range (red lines)

sider how their weight has changed over the past 4 weeks rather than in a single weigh-in. Weight fluctuations are natural and can occur due to physiological factors (e.g., premenstrual phase) as well as variations in energy balance. If weight increases over 1 or 2 weeks, the patient should not be concerned because the weight variation may be transient and secondary to changes in hydration status. However, if a weight gain trend over 4 weeks is evident, the patient should implement their action plan without delay.

19.4.5 Adopting Eating Habits for Weight Maintenance

The specific strategies that the therapist should suggest for the patient to maintain weight depend on the trend in their weight over the previous 4 weeks. If the patient's weight appears stable, as is often the case, no changes to the energy balance are necessary. If, however, the patient's weight displays a decreasing trend, and they have agreed to start the maintenance phase, the calorie intake should be increased based on the amount of weight lost (e.g., an increase of 500 kcal per day for a loss of 2 kg in 4 weeks, as 1 kg of weight loss corresponds to approximately an energy deficit of about 7,000 kcal).

Furthermore, the therapist should advise the patient to maintain the same nutritional composition as the dietary plan adopted during weight loss (see Chap. 12). However, if a patient has lost weight by incorporating a low percentage of proteins (e.g., less than 25%) but a relatively high proportion of carbohydrates, the therapist should inform them about the findings of a large randomized controlled trial that observed better weight maintenance with a high-protein, low-glycaemic index, and moderate-fat content ad libitum diet [10]. Based on these results, patients should increase protein intake and limit foods with a high glycaemic index. The therapist should also remind the patient to maintain the eating habits they have adopted, especially eating regularly (i.e., three meals and two snacks per day) and following a flexible and healthy dietary plan.

19.4.6 Exercising for Weight Maintenance

Studies have extensively confirmed that regular physical activity is associated with long-term weight maintenance [11]. However, how much exercise is necessary, and what specific types of exercise are more effective than others for maintaining lost weight? One answer to this question comes from data related to participants in the NWCR. That indicates that individuals who have succeeded in maintaining lost weight have engaged in higher levels of physical activity (burning an average of approximately 2,600 kcal/week, equivalent to ~60–75 minutes per day of moderate-intensity activity, such as brisk walking) compared to the traditional goal recommended by physicians for weight control (1,000 kcal/week) [12]. Walking was the preferred activity among NWCR participants, but approximately 29% also reported engaging in some form of resistance training. Although resistance training is not mandatory for successful weight maintenance, it can enhance daily energy expenditure by promoting an increase in muscle mass. That said, about 92% of NWCR participants who reported engaging in resistance training also participated in other types of physical activity [12].

The quantity and type of exercise practiced by those who succeeded in the NWCR are similar to those recommended by CBT for BED (see Chap. 8). For this reason, the therapist should encourage the patient to continue with the exercise plan adopted during the weight-loss phase if it is sufficiently intensive (e.g., at least 10,000 steps per day). Otherwise, the patient should be encouraged to gradually increase their physical activity to achieve similar energy expenditure, which will enhance their ability to maintain lost weight in the long term.

19.4.7 Developing a Weight Maintenance Mindset

Cognitive processes play a crucial role in a patient's ability to stick with behaviours necessary for weight maintenance. Our research has indicated that 3 years after treatment, patients who were satisfied with the results or confident in their ability to control weight without further professional assistance were more likely to succeed in long-term weight maintenance [13]. This finding highlights the importance of a construct similar to the concept of self-efficacy, which is associated with increased adherence to weight management. It is therefore surprising that cognitive strategies are not more commonly utilized in traditional weight-management programmes.

Assuming that self-efficacy might be one reason for their partial effectiveness, the Maintenance Preparation module includes specific procedures designed to help the patient develop a "weight-maintenance mindset". The first step in this process is to collaboratively create a list of the patient's reasons for maintaining their current weight. To assist in making this list, the therapist should encourage the patient to focus on four domains of their life: physical health, psychological well-being, interpersonal relationships, and work performance, and consider both short- and long-term perspectives. The patient should be encouraged to consult this list when their motivation begins to waver to restore their focus on weight control.

The therapist should encourage the patient to maintain the eating and physical activity habits that led to these positive changes, as they will be necessary for long-term success. In most cases, these are already established and do not require significant cognitive effort. However, the patient should also be cautioned against persistently reverting to old lifestyle habits. They should be informed that the more consistently a person practices a behaviour, the more likely it is to become automatic and easy to implement. In contrast, the opposite occurs when one is inattentive and reverts to old dysfunctional habits. It can be helpful to compare eating control to physical training when explaining this concept: the more a person trains their muscles, the less effort it takes, while regaining previous fitness levels after taking a break from exercising will require a lot of hard work.

Another strategy we recommend to patients is to adopt a weight-maintenance mindset focused on their personal motivations for weight maintenance. They should be encouraged to practice the following cognitive skills they learned during the weight-loss phase:

- Mentally planning when, what, and where to eat at the beginning of the day.
- Eating consciously: appreciating the smell and taste of food, and sticking to the eating plan without being influenced by external (e.g., sight of food, events) or internal (e.g., desires, need for gratification, hunger, thoughts about food, mood changes) factors that may negatively impact their adherence to the plan.
- Giving themselves cognitive credits each week if their weight remained within the maintenance range, using phrases like the following: "*I did well,*" "*I'm doing great,*" *and* "*I can do this.*" Regular use of cognitive credits can help the patient reduce the frustration associated with maintaining a long-term weight-control-oriented lifestyle, and bolster their confidence in their ability to control weight.
- Using the proactive problem-solving procedure to address events that could impact eating.
- Deploying the "things to say and do" procedure to address mood changes, urges to overeat, and cravings for high-calorie foods.
- Displacing the eating-disorder mindset when thoughts arise that may lead to "backsliding", to help them get back on track (see Sect. 18.2.3)

19.5 Drawing Up the Maintenance Plan

Patients need to be well prepared to face the maintenance period (i.e., Step Three of the treatment). To this end, the last thing to accomplish is to develop a personalized written maintenance plan collaboratively. This will contain individualized advice on which residual features of BED and weight maintenance (if indicated) to address and, at the same time, how to minimize the risk of relapse (e.g., reminders on how to deal with triggers and setbacks). The template shown in Table 19.2 may be modified for this purpose. The patient should be given a copy of their maintenance plan, and the therapist invite them to read it periodically so that they can refer to it systematically.

Table 19.2 Maintenance plan template

MAINTENANCE PLAN FOR	
Focus Areas	What to Do
Binge-eating episodes	• Analyze binge episodes, if they arise, to identify triggers (eating too little; going too long without eating; breaking a dietary rule; drinking alcohol, which promotes disinhibition; life events) and address them. • Practice the proactive problem-solving procedure to manage events influencing eating. • Immediately decentre from the BED mindset (do the opposite). • Do not view lapses as relapses, but as opportunities to improve eating control (no black-and-white thinking). • Do not jump to worst-case scenario: keep calm, analyze the reasons for the setback, and use the proactive problem-solving procedure to get back on track immediately.
Dysfunctional dieting	• Eat regularly (3 meals + 2 snacks and nothing in between) - Adopt a flexible and healthy attitude to eating. - Avoid extreme and rigid dietary rules.
Active lifestyle	• Reduce sedentary activities, increase daily step count, improve physical fitness.
Events, moods, and eating	• Practice proactive problem-solving to manage events influencing eating. • Work on enhancing the importance of other rewarding activities. • Use healthy coping strategies to deal with mood intolerance (predict and prevent the triggering event, perform a cognitive assessment of events, accept emotions, use functional mood-modulation behaviours).
Overvaluation of shape and weight, and internalized weight stigma	• Stay vigilant against shape checking (e.g., frequent use of the mirror, inappropriate checking of clothing, pinching fat folds, comparison checks); consider whether the information this gives you is accurate and helpful. • Do not avoid looking at your body. If it happens, try to be more body-aware (e.g., change clothes, get a massage). • Use the mirror carefully. • Only weigh yourself once a week, and do not attempt to interpret a single reading. • Avoid judging yourself solely based on your weight and body shape: give yourself cognitive credits for things you have done well. Avoid critics for your weight, shape and eating control. • Maintain and develop other interests (e.g., ...)

(continued)

Table 19.2 (continued)

MAINTENANCE PLAN FOR	
Focus Areas	What to Do
Weight goals and primary goals	• Remember the benefits of your current weight and the risks of wanting to lose additional weight (refer to your pros and cons table). • Strive for any remaining primary goals without trying to lose weight. • Practice accepting the reasonable and healthy weight you have achieved.
Weight maintenance	• Weigh yourself once a week and interpret weight variations over a 4-week span. • Maintain weight within a range of between……. to……. • If weight goes above ……. kg, go into "danger" mode: – Resume real-time monitoring. – Reduce your daily intake by 500 kcal until your weight returns to the maintenance range (over a 4-week span), then adjust your meal plan for weight maintenance. – Address the underlying causes using the proactive problem-solving procedure. • Train your weight maintenance mindset: – Read your weight-maintenance plan every week. – Mentally plan when, where, and what to eat every day – Address the urge to eat unplanned foods using the "things to say and do" procedure. – Use proactive problem-solving to address circumstances, events (e.g., holidays, social occasions, periods of stress, illnesses), and mood changes that could negatively affect eating behaviour.

References

1. Dalle Grave R, Sartirana M, El Ghoch M, Calugi S. Treating obesity with personalized cognitive behavioral therapy. Cham: Springer; 2018.
2. Klem ML, Wing RR, McGuire MT, Seagle HM, Hill JO. A descriptive study of individuals successful at long-term maintenance of substantial weight loss. Am J Clin Nutr. 1997;66(2):239–46. https://doi.org/10.1093/ajcn/66.2.239.
3. Keesey RE, Hirvonen MD. Body weight set-points: determination and adjustment. J Nutr. 1997;127(9):1875s–83s. https://doi.org/10.1093/jn/127.9.1875S.
4. Qasim A, Turcotte M, de Souza RJ, Samaan MC, Champredon D, Dushoff J, et al. On the origin of obesity: identifying the biological, environmental and cultural drivers of genetic risk among human populations. Obes Rev. 2018;19(2):121–49. https://doi.org/10.1111/obr.12625.
5. Calugi S, Marchesini G, El Ghoch M, Gavasso I, Dalle GR. The influence of weight-loss expectations on weight loss and of weight-loss satisfaction on weight maintenance in severe obesity. J Acad Nutr Diet. 2017;117(1):32–8. https://doi.org/10.1016/j.jand.2016.09.001.
6. Calugi S, Marchesini G, El Ghoch M, Gavasso I, Dalle GR. The association between weight maintenance and session-by-session diet adherence, weight loss and weight-loss satisfaction. Eat Weight Disord. 2020;25(1):127–33. https://doi.org/10.1007/s40519-018-0528-8.
7. Pacanowski CR, Linde JA, Neumark-Sztainer D. Self-weighing: helpful or harmful for psychological well-being? A review of the literature. Curr Obes Rep. 2015;4(1):65–72. https://doi.org/10.1007/s13679-015-0142-2.
8. McGuire MT, Wing RR, Klem ML, Hill JO. Behavioral strategies of individuals who have maintained long-term weight losses. Obes Res. 1999;7(4):334–41. https://doi.org/10.1002/j.1550-8528.1999.tb00416.x.

9. Cooper Z, Fairburn CG, Hawker DM. Cognitive-behavioral treatment of obesity: a clinician's guide. Guilford Press; 2003.
10. Larsen TM, Dalskov SM, van Baak M, Jebb SA, Papadaki A, Pfeiffer AF, et al. Diets with high or low protein content and glycemic index for weight-loss maintenance. N Engl J Med. 2010;363(22):2102–13. https://doi.org/10.1056/NEJMoa1007137.
11. Pronk NP, Wing RR. Physical activity and long-term maintenance of weight loss. Obes Res. 1994;2(6):587–99. https://doi.org/10.1002/j.1550-8528.1994.tb00110.x.
12. Catenacci VA, Ogden LG, Stuht J, Phelan S, Wing RR, Hill JO, et al. Physical activity patterns in the National Weight Control Registry. Obesity. 2008;16(1):153–61. https://doi.org/10.1038/oby.2007.6.
13. Dalle Grave R, Melchionda N, Calugi S, Centis E, Tufano A, Fatati G, et al. Continuous care in the treatment of obesity: an observational multicentre study. J Intern Med. 2005;258(3):265–73. https://doi.org/10.1111/j.1365-2796.2005.01524.x.

20 Preventing Relapse

Abstract

Step Three of cognitive behaviour therapy (CBT) for binge-eating disorder (BED) lasts 48 weeks, with 12 sessions delivered at 4-week intervals in patients who addressed the Healthy Weight Loss module in Step Two of the tretment, that are reduced to 12 weeks, with 3 sessions every 4 weeks, in all the other patients. The focus of the sessions is on assessing both the eating-disorder psychopathology and progress in weight maintenance over the last 4 weeks. The session begins by reviewing how the patient has implemented the maintenance plan, to identify the features of BED and difficulties in weight maintenance that the patient will need to tackle. The need for weekly weighing should be reiterated. In this phase, it is essential to emphasize to the patient that their attitude toward any setback is crucial in determining what will happen next. Specifically, they are encouraged not to view any setback (e.g., a binge episode) as a "relapse." They are also helped to identify and address situations that increase the risk of weight regain and implement an action plan that promptly addresses it. For a patient who wants to lose weight in the future, the therapist should suggest careful consideration of their reasons, and the potential risks involved. Finally, at the conclusion of Step Three, the patient should be explicitly educated on self-efficacy, and reassured of the fact that they now have all the tools they need to maintain weight on their own and deal with any situation that might otherwise lead to relapse.

Step Three of the treatment lasts 48 weeks and includes 12 sessions at 4-week intervals. The objectives of this phase are the following:

- Reviewing how the maintenance plan is being implemented
- Preventing a lapse (e.g., a binge-eating episode) from turning into a relapse
- Identifying and addressing situations that increase the risk of weight regain
- Addressing the possibility of weight regain

R. Dalle Grave et al., *Cognitive Behavior Therapy for Binge Eating Disorder*,
https://doi.org/10.1007/978-3-031-71456-6_20

- Weighing up potential future weight-loss attempts
- Winding up the treatment

During the sessions in this Step, the progress of the eating disorder and weight maintenance should be assessed by discussing the challenges and achievements of the past 4 weeks with the patient. In particular, the patient should be assisted in reviewing whether they have successfully followed the maintenance plan and how they managed any setbacks that may have occurred.

20.1 Reviewing Implementation of the Maintenance Plan

The session should begin with a thorough review of how the patient has implemented the maintenance plan. The plan should be examined point by point, aiming to identify any BED features or difficulties in weight maintenance that the patient should continue to work on. The need for weekly weighing should be reiterated. The therapist should assess whether to continue filling in the EPCL-BED based on the patient's ability to identify and manage setbacks. Any setbacks should be discussed in detail, and the patient's strategies should be reviewed and potentially improved. Finally, if necessary, the maintenance plan should be revised to address any new triggers or situations that may have emerged.

20.2 Preventing a Lapse Becoming a Relapse

In this phase, it is important to emphasize to the patient that their attitude towards any setback is crucial in determining what will happen next. Specifically, they are encouraged not to view any slip (e.g., a binge-eating episode) as a relapse—a passive and hopeless attitude that is highly likely to lead to loss of all the benefits achieved by the treatment. Instead, the patient should identify any setback as a temporary lapse, a strategy that should make them more inclined to resolve the problem successfully. In particular, the therapist should discuss the following concepts with the patient [1, 2]:

- The need to have realistic expectations regarding eating because it is almost impossible to eat healthily on every occasion.
- The importance of immediately recognizing high-risk situations and applying appropriate responses to forestall a lapse (e.g., planning ahead, eating consciously, self-talk, proactive problem-solving, and distancing from problematic thoughts)
- The importance of reacting constructively if a binge occurs, conducting a binge-eating analysis (see Sect. 13.5.1), and immediately getting back on track to prevent a lapse from turning into a relapse.
- The importance of analyzing and addressing the underlying motives of the lapse using the proactive problem-solving procedure.

20.3 Identifying and Addressing Situations That Increase the Risk of Weight Regain

Patients who lost weight in Step Two of the treatment should be educated on the situations that put them at high risk of weight regain. These can be divided into three main categories [3, 4]: (i) high-risk circumstances, (ii) problematic behaviours, and (iii) dysfunctional thoughts. The patient should be taught to recognize and address these situations appropriately. For example, to cope with high-risk circumstances (e.g., vacations, forced periods of inactivity, illness), the patient should implement two main strategies:

1. Have an action plan ready.
2. Evaluate the pros and cons of preventing weight gain or suspending weight maintenance for a limited period and then take compensatory action once the risk has passed.

Common behaviours that increase the risk of weight regain include dysregulated eating, eating high-fat and high-calorie foods in general or overeating during stress, reducing overall exercise, overeating during holidays, and overeating in social situations. Each of these problematic behaviours should be addressed through the proactive problem-solving procedure.

Finally, various problematic thoughts can lead to abandoning eating and physical activity control habits and result in weight regain, but the two most common are as follows [4]:

1. *Dysfunctional reactions to weight regain*. Examples include abandoning weekly weighing ("ostrich" thinking), hoping the problem will resolve on its own ("vain hope" thinking), and giving up any attempt to control weight ("all-or-nothing" thinking).
2. *False confidence*. Example: "*I can eat whatever I want without gaining weight.*" This attitude tends to develop when a person has not observed weight gain after a brief period of dysregulated eating. Unfortunately, it is inevitable that maintaining a positive energy balance for an extended period of time will lead to weight gain.

To address problematic thoughts and attitudes, the therapist should encourage the patient to apply the procedures described in the Setbacks and Mindsets module (Chap. 18).

20.4 Addressing Weight Regain

Weight maintenance requires balancing calorie intake and energy expenditure. Although the role of physical exercise in weight maintenance should not be underestimated, controlling energy intake is the most important aspect of maintaining this balance. However, weight regain commonly results from changes in energy intake, energy expenditure, or both. The therapist should inform the patient that if weight regain occurs, they should immediately implement an action plan that includes the following steps [3]:

- Identify the type of weight change: is it a sudden jump or a trend?
- Identify the reason for weight regain (in terms of energy balance): is it due to an increase in energy intake (more common), a decrease in energy expenditure, or both?
- Identify the underlying causes: is it due to poor management of high-risk periods (e.g., holidays, work stress, illness), the adoption of problematic behaviours (e.g., eating junk food, overeating in social situations, snacking, binge episodes, excessive alcohol consumption), or the effect of dysfunctional thoughts (e.g., dysfunctional reaction to weight regain or false confidence)?
- Design and implement an action plan to react constructively to weight regain based on why it occurred. Reduce calorie intake and/or increase energy expenditure to create a negative energy balance of 500 kcal/day until the weight returns to the weight-maintenance range. Once this happens, adjust calorie intake and/or energy expenditure back to previous weight-maintenance levels.
- Design and implement a plan to address underlying causes. Use the proactive problem-solving procedure.

The therapist should also suggest that the patient use the proactive problem-solving procedure in the event of three possible scenarios:

1. Weight gain (e.g., after returning from vacation, during pregnancy, or after a period of inactivity due to illness)
2. A situation that might increase the risk of weight regain (e.g., quitting smoking, retiring, changing jobs, experiencing a family crisis, a hospital stay, entering menopause)
3. A situation in which it is not possible to do weekly weighing (e.g., because the scales are broken or being in a location for a long time where it is not possible to do so).

The patient should be encouraged to explore these potential scenarios and find effective solutions in advance. During these sessions, the therapist–patient interaction style should begin to change, becoming more future-oriented and encouraging the patient to resolve problems independently.

20.5 Weighing Up Potential Future Weight-loss Attempts

For a patient who wants to lose weight in the future, the therapist should suggest careful consideration of the reasons and potential risks involved. For example, will further weight loss truly achieve the desired result? What are the chances that attempting a very low-energy diet will increase the risk of binge-eating episodes and/or disruptions to the habits necessary for healthy weight maintenance? Even if determined to undertake another weight-loss attempt, they should be encouraged to wait for an appropriate period (i.e., at least 48 weeks), allowing them the opportunity to learn and practice weight-maintenance skills, as these will be necessary for long-term recovery.

20.6 Winding Up the Treatment

Towards the end of Step Three, the patient should be explicitly instructed on self-efficacy [5]. They should be reassured that they now have all the tools they need to maintain weight on their own and prevent relapse into the eating disorder. They should be told that it is time to apply the procedures learned during the treatment without the therapist's supervision. The therapist should do their best to ensure the treatment ends well, and congratulate the patient on the results, attributing their success to their dedication and capabilities. Then, the patient should be asked how they feel about the treatment ending, and encouraged to continue applying the following key procedures:

Reviewing the maintenance plan periodically
Weighing themselves weekly and interpreting any changes appropriately
Addressing setbacks and BED mindset reactivation
Maintaining the dietary and exercise habits necessary for weight control
Keeping the weight-maintenance mindset active at all times

Vignette

The patient, a 45-year-old divorced biologist who had achieved a weight loss of 12 kg and remission from binge-eating episodes at the end of the first 24 weeks of treatment, began Step Three of the treatment without any reluctance because she was satisfied with both the weight loss and the improvement in her control over eating and physical fitness. During maintenance, however, she experienced several episodes of weight regain, as she had recurring binge-eating episodes during the premenstrual phase. Nevertheless, by implementing her personal action plan, she was always able to lose the weight she had regained and return to the weight-maintenance range. Using the proactive problem-solving procedure, she discovered that, by avoiding scheduling stressful commitments, not drinking alcohol, and planning meals and snacks with high-quality complex carbohydrates during the premenstrual phase, she could reduce and cope with the cravings for sweet things she usually experienced and forestall binge-eating episodes.

References

1. Dalle Grave R, Calugi S. Cognitive behavior therapy for adolescents with eating disorders. New York: Guilford Press; 2020.
2. Fairburn CG. Cognitive behavior therapy and eating disorders. New York: Guilford Press; 2008.
3. Cooper Z, Fairburn CG. A new cognitive behavioural approach to the treatment of obesity. Behav Res Ther. 2001;39(5):499–511.
4. Dalle Grave R, Sartirana M, El Ghoch M, Calugi S. Treating obesity with personalized cognitive behavioral therapy. Cham: Springer; 2018.
5. Bandura A. Social foundations of thought and action: a social cognitive theory. Englewood Cliffs: Prentice-Hall; 1986.

Appendix 1 – Monitoring Record

During treatment, it is essential that you record everything that you eat or drink and what is going on at the time. We call this "self-monitoring". Its purpose is two-fold: first, it provides a detailed picture of how you eat, thereby bringing to your attention and that of your therapist the exact nature of your eating problem; and second, by making you more aware of what you are doing at the very time that you are doing it, self-monitoring helps you change behaviours which may previously have seemed automatic and beyond your control. Accurate "real-time" monitoring is central to treatment. It will help you change.

At first, writing down everything that you eat may be irritating and inconvenient, but soon, it will become second nature and of obvious value. We have yet to encounter anyone whose lifestyle made monitoring impossible. Regard it as a challenge,

Look at the sample monitoring record to see how to monitor. A new record (or records) should be started each day.

In **Column 1**, write down the times you ate or drank anything.

In **Column 2**, report the foods and drinks consumed. Calories should not be recorded; you should write down a simple (non-technical) description of what you ate or drank. Each item should be written down as soon as possible after consumption. Recalling what you ate or drank some hours afterward will not work since it will not help you change your behaviour at the time. If you are to record this way, you must carry your monitoring sheets with you. It does not matter if your records are messy or the writing or spelling is bad. The important thing is that you record everything you eat or drink as soon as possible afterward. Episodes of eating that you view as meals should be identified with brackets. Snacks and other episodes of eating should not be bracketed.

In **Column 3**, report where you consumed the food. If this happens at home, the room must be specified.

In **Column 4**, indicate with an asterisk each eating episode (each food) that you consider excessive at the time. This is your judgement, regardless of what anyone else might think. It is essential to record all the foods eaten during a binge-eating episode, and identify them as a chain of asterisks. As always, you need to be honest, with no embarrassment or fear of being judged. In order to overcome your binge eating, you need to accurately record events as they happen.

R. Dalle Grave et al., *Cognitive Behavior Therapy for Binge Eating Disorder*,
https://doi.org/10.1007/978-3-031-71456-6

Column 5 will be used in various ways during treatment. For the moment it should be used as a diary to record the events, thoughts, and feelings about what you ate. For example, if an argument precipitated a binge or led you not to eat, you should note that down. Try to write a brief comment every time you eat, recording your thoughts and feelings about what you ate.

You may want to record other important events or circumstances in this column, even if they had no effect on your eating. The last column should also record your weight (and your thoughts about it) each time you weigh yourself.

The **Steps** row should be used to report daily steps measured with a pedometer.

The **Formal Exercise** tow should be used to report the type and minutes of formal exercise (i.e., physical activity that requires effort and increases heart and breathing rates, such as swimming, tennis, running) During formal physical exercise, the pedometer should be removed.

Every treatment session will include a detailed review of your latest monitoring records. You should, therefore, remember to bring them with you! (Fig. A1.1)

Day ____________________ **Date** ____________________

Time	**Food and drink consumed**	**Place**	*	**Comments**
Steps		Number:		
Formal exercise		Type:		Minutes:

Fig. A1.1 The monitoring record

Appendix 2 – Weight Graph (Fig. A2.1)

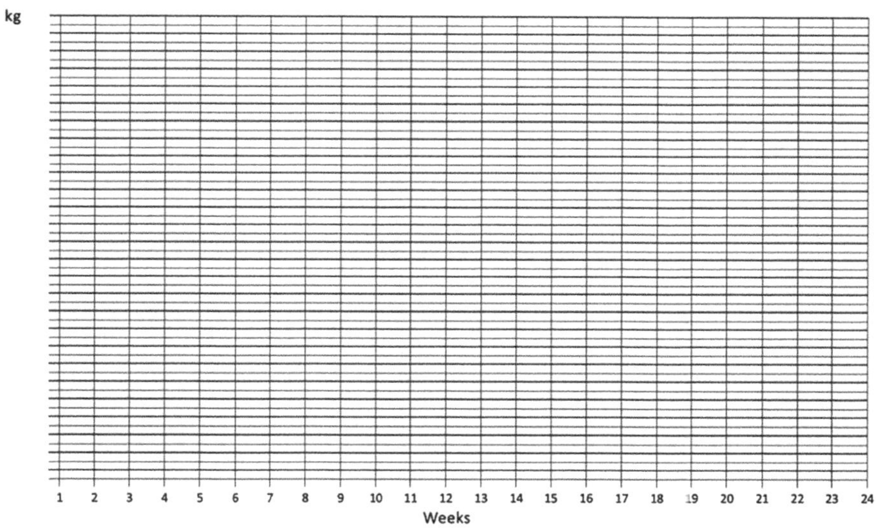

Fig. A2.1 The weight graph

R. Dalle Grave et al., *Cognitive Behavior Therapy for Binge Eating Disorder*, https://doi.org/10.1007/978-3-031-71456-6

Appendix 3 – Eating Problem Checklist for Binge-Eating Disorder (EPCL-BED)

The EPCL-BED (Table A3.1) is a 14-item self-report measure designed to assess eating-disorder behaviours and psychopathology, session by session, in patients

Table A3.1 Eating Problem Check List for Binge-Eating Disorder (EPCL-BEDL)

Eating Problem Check List for Binge-Eating Disorder (EPCL-BEDL)

INSTRUCTIONS: The following questions are concerned with the past seven days only. Please read each question carefully. Please answer all the questions. Thank you.

In the past seven days... *(indicate the number of times that this has occurred in the box on the right)*	**No. of episodes**
Have you eaten a large amount of food with a sense of having lost control (i.e. an objective binge-eating episode)?	
Have you eaten a not large amount of food with a sense of having lost control (i.e. a subjective binge-eating episode)?	
Have you eaten between meals and snacks?	
Have you eaten more than you planned at meals and snacks?	
Have you drunk too much alcohol?	
Have you weighed yourself?	

In the past seven days, how often... *(tick which box is true for you)*	**0 Never**	**1 Rarely**	**2 Sometimes**	**3 Often**	**4 Always**
Have events and associated mood changes influenced your eating?					
Have food environmental stimuli influenced your eating?					
Have you tried to adopt extreme and rigid dietary rules to control your weight and/or body shape?					
Have you checked your shape (e.g. looking at parts of your body in the mirror; measuring the circumference of parts of your body; compared your body shape with that of other people)?					
Have you avoided your body (e.g. avoided weighing, avoided particular clothes, avoided looking at your body)?					
Have you been concerned about your weight?					
Have you been concerned about your shape?					
Have you been concerned about your eating control?					

R. Dalle Grave et al., *Cognitive Behavior Therapy for Binge Eating Disorder*,
https://doi.org/10.1007/978-3-031-71456-6

with binge-eating disorders. It is focused on the past 7 days. The 14 items cover the principal behaviours and attitudes of eating-disorder psychopathology in people with binge-eating disorder. It is quick and easy to complete, and enables therapist and patient to assess, through a review of each single item score, any changes in specific expressions of binge-eating disorder psychopathology at weekly intervals. It aids identification of improvement and/or deterioration, and allows the treatment to be focused on specific expressions of an individual's eating-disorder psychopathology.

In our clinical practice, we find it useful to review and discuss the single-item EPCL-BED scores carefully with the patient on a weekly basis (after the collaborative weighing procedure) carefully. This review, if associated with a review of the last 7 days' monitoring records, helps to highlight—when there is a variation of at least 1 point in one or more items of the EPCL-BED—the changes that patients have made over the week, and identify the behavioural and cognitive expressions of their eating-disorder psychopathology to be addressed.

In addition, recording EPCL-BED data on a summary spreadsheet (Table A3.2) weekly makes it possible to observe whether modification of certain behaviours (e.g., adopting regular eating, reducing dietary restraint, weekly weighing, and/or interrupting dysfunctional body checking) is associated with a reduction in concerns about eating, shape, and weight over time—one of the primary goals and theoretical underpinnings of CBT for binge-eating disorder.

The EPCL and its items are under copyright. However, it is freely available for non-commercial research use only and no permission need be sought.

Table A3.2 Weekly Changes Summary Spreadsheet

Date																								
Week																								
Body weight (kg)																								
Objective binge eating[1]																								
Eating between meals and snacks[1]																								
Eating more than planned[1]																								
Drinking too much alcohol[1]																								
Weight checking[1]																								
Events, mood and eating[2]																								
Environmental stimuli[2]																								
Extreme and rigid diet[2]																								
Body shape checking[2]																								
Body avoidance[2]																								
Weight concern[2]																								
Body shape concern [2]																								
Eating concern [2]																								

[1]number of episodes in the last 7 days

[2]0 = never, 1 = rarely, 2 = sometimes, 3 = often, 4 = always

Appendix 4 –The Weight-Loss Obstacles Questionnaire

Instructions: The following questions refer to the past seven days only. Please read each question carefully. Please answer all the questions.

PROCEDURES

1. Did you fill in your Monitoring Records every day? ☐ yes ☐ no
If not, how many days did you miss? ________ What was the reason?

____
____
____

2. Did you count calories every day? ☐ yes ☐ no
If not, how many days did you miss? ________ What was the reason?

____
____
____

3. Did you do your physical activity every day? ☐ yes ☐ no
If not, how many days did you miss? ________ What was the reason?

____
____
____

4. Did you use a step counter every day? ☐ yes ☐ no
If not, how many days did you miss? ________ What was the reason?

____
____
____

5. Did you check your weight once a week? ☐ yes ☐ no
If not, how many days did you check your weight? ________ What was the reason?

____
____
____

6. Did you stick to your calorie limit every day? ☐ yes ☐ no
If not, how many days did you go over the limit? ________ What was the reason?

____
____
____

7. Did you do at least 10,000 steps every day? ☐ yes ☐ no
If not, how many days did you miss? ________ What was the reason?

____
____
____

R. Dalle Grave et al., *Cognitive Behavior Therapy for Binge Eating Disorder*,
https://doi.org/10.1007/978-3-031-71456-6

BEHAVIOURS

8. Did you eat between meals? ☐ yes ☐ no

If yes, how many times did you eat between meals? ________ What was the reason?

____

____

____

9. Did you overeat at mealtimes? ☐ yes ☐ no

If so, how many times? ________ What was the reason?

____

____

____

10. Did you skip any meals? ☐ yes ☐ no

If so, how many times? ________ What was the reason?

____

____

____

11. Did you have any episodes of binge eating (i.e., being unable to stop yourself eating a large amount of food)? ☐ yes ☐ no

If so, how many times? ________ What was the reason?

____

____

____

12. Did you eat during the night? ☐ yes ☐ no

If so, how many times? ________ What was the reason?

____

____

____

13. Did you avoid eating certain food groups on some days? ☐ yes ☐ no

If so, how many times? ________ What was the reason?

____

____

____

14. Did you drink too much alcohol? ☐ yes ☐ no

If so, how many times? ________ What was the reason?

____

____

____

ATTITUDES

15. How satisfied are you with your weight loss so far?

0 1 2 3 4 5 6 7 8 9 10
Not at all Extremely

16. How able do you think you are to lose weight?

0 1 2 3 4 5 6 7 8 9 10
Not at all Extremely

17. How motivated are you to lose weight?

0 1 2 3 4 5 6 7 8 9 10
Not at all Extremely

SOCIAL SUPPORT

How often have you received support from significant others?

18. In times of crisis

0 1 2 3 4 5 6 7 8 9 10
Never Always

19. In creating an environment that facilitates change

0 1 2 3 4 5 6 7 8 9 10
Never Always

20. In applying the programme procedures

0 1 2 3 4 5 6 7 8 9 10
Never Always

How often have you received criticism from significant others?

21. On your body weight

0 1 2 3 4 5 6 7 8 9 10
Never Always

22. On your eating behaviour

0 1 2 3 4 5 6 7 8 9 10
Never Always

23. On your level of physical activity

0 1 2 3 4 5 6 7 8 9 10
Never Always

Appendix 5 – Weight Goals and Primary Goals Questionnaire

Questions on your weight goal:

1. What is your dream weight (the weight you would reach in an ideal world, even though you understand that this is probably unattainable)?

   ____

2. What is your desired weight (the weight you think you should and probably will achieve during the treatment)? ___________
3. What is your acceptable weight (the highest weight you think you would be able to accept)?

   ____

Questions on your desired weight (the weight you wrote in question 2):

4. In the past, was your desired weight different?

   ☐ yes ☐ no

   If so, why? ____

5. How long have you been at your desired weight in your life?
   - ☐ Less than 1 year
   - ☐ Between 1 and 3 years
   - ☐ Between 3 and 5 years
   - ☐ More than 5 years

6. How hard do you think it will be to remain at your desired weight?

   Very A lot A little Not very

7. How important is it for you to achieve your desired weight?

   Very A lot A little Not very

8. How would you feel if you did not reach your desired weight?

____

____

R. Dalle Grave et al., *Cognitive Behavior Therapy for Binge Eating Disorder*,
https://doi.org/10.1007/978-3-031-71456-6

Questions on your primary reasons for losing weight:

Instructions: Please put an X in the box you think most appropriate for each statement.

1 = Totally disagree; **2** = Disagree; **3** = Slightly disagree;

4 = Slightly agree; **5** = Agree; **6** = Totally agree

9. Why do you want to reach your desired weight?

	1	2	3	4	5	6
To improve physical appearance						
To reduce the size of some parts of your body						
To reducing clothing size						
To have a greater choice of clothes						
To reach the weight advised by the doctor						
To go back to the weight you were at an important time in your life						
To go back to the weight you achieved in a previous weight-loss attempt						
To reach your ideal weight, according to the ideal weight table						
To have the same weight as other people your age						
To have the same weight as friends or family members						
To have the same weight as famous people						
To improve your health						
To improve your physical fitness						
To improve the quality of your free time						
To improve your sex life						
To be more sexually attractive to others						
To get attention or approval from others						
To get a promotion						
To get a new job						
To improve your social life						
To prevent bias against people with overweight or obesity						
To improve your interpersonal relationships						
To improve your self-esteem						
To feel better psychologically						
To be able to have a baby						
To be around for your children						

Of the primary reasons you scored "5" or "6" in question 9:

10. Which is the most important? ______________________________

11. Which necessarily require weight loss? ______________________________

12. Which do not necessarily require weight loss? ______________________________

13. How would it feel if you did not achieve these goals? ______________________________

The manufacturer's authorised representative in the EU is Springer Nature Customer Service Centre GmbH, Europaplatz 3, 69115 Heidelberg, Germany. If you have any concerns regarding our products, please contact ProductSafety@springernature.com

Printed and bound by CPI Group (UK) Ltd, Croydon, CR0 4YY
01/10/2026
02225859-0005